EXTERNAL EAR MALFORMATIONS: EPIDEMIOLOGY, GENETICS, AND NATURAL HISTORY

BOOKS PUBLISHED BY ALAN R. LISS, INC.
FOR THE NATIONAL FOUNDATION

Birth Defects Compendium, Second Edition, Daniel Bergsma, *Editor*

BIRTH DEFECTS: ORIGINAL ARTICLE SERIES
1979 — Volume XV

No. 1 **Sex Chromosome Aneuploidy: Prospective Studies on Children,** Arthur Robinson, Herbert A. Lubs, and Daniel Bergsma, *Editors*

No. 2 **Genetic Counseling: Facts, Values, and Norms,** Alexander M. Capron, Marc Lappé, Robert F. Murray, Jr., Tabitha M. Powledge, Sumner B. Twiss, and Daniel Bergsma, *Editors*

No. 3 **Recent Advances in the Developmental Biology of Central Nervous System Malformation,** Ntinos C. Myrianthopoulos and Daniel Bergsma, *Editors*

No. 4 **Continuous Transcutaneous Blood Gas Monitoring,** A. Huch, R. Huch, and J. Lucey, *Editors*

No. 5 **Annual Review of Birth Defects, 1978,** Proceedings of the 1978 San Francisco Birth Defects Conference. Published in 3 volumes:

    5A **Diagnostic Approaches to the Malformed Fetus, Abortus, Stillborn, and Deceased Newborn,** Mitchell S. Golbus and Bryan D. Hall, *Editors*

    5B **Penetrance and Variability in Malformation Syndromes,** James J. O'Donnell and Bryan D. Hall, *Editors*

    5C **Risks, Communication, and Decision Making in Genetic Counseling,** Charles J. Epstein, Cynthia J.R. Curry, Seymour Packman, Sanford Sherman, and Bryan D. Hall, *Editors*

No. 6 **Dermatoglyphics — Fifty Years Later,** Wladimir Wertelecki and Chris C. Plato, *Editors*

No. 7 **Newborn Behavioral Organization: Nursing Research and Implications,** Gene C. Anderson and Beverly Raff, *Editors*

No. 8 **Developmental Aspects of Craniofacial Dysmorphology,** Michael Melnick and Ronald Jorgenson, *Editors*

No. 9 **External Ear Malformations: Epidemiology, Genetics, and Natural History,** *by* Michael Melnick and Ntinos C. Myrianthopoulos

See pages 139–140 for other volumes in this series published by Alan R. Liss, Inc.

The National Foundation–March of Dimes
Birth Defects: Original Article Series, Volume XV, Number 9, 1979

EXTERNAL EAR MALFORMATIONS: EPIDEMIOLOGY, GENETICS, AND NATURAL HISTORY

Michael Melnick, DDS, PhD
Laboratory for Developmental Biology
Andrus Gerontology Center
University of Southern California
Los Angeles, California
and
Ntinos C. Myrianthopoulos, PhD
Developmental Neurology Branch
National Institute of Neurological and Communicative
Disorders and Stroke
National Institutes of Health
Bethesda, Maryland

Natalie W. Paul
Associate Editor – The National Foundation

ALAN R. LISS, INC., NEW YORK

To enhance medical communication in the birth defects field, The National Foundation publishes the *Birth Defects Compendium (Second Edition)*, an *Original Article Series, Syndrome Identification,* a *Reprint Series,* and provides a series of films and related brochures.

Further information can be obtained from:

The National Foundation
Professional Education Division
1275 Mamaroneck Avenue
White Plains, New York 10605

Published by:

Alan R. Liss, Inc.
150 Fifth Avenue
New York, New York 10011

Copyright © 1979 by The National Foundation

All rights reserved. No part of this publication may be reproduced or transmitted in any form or by any means, electronic or mechanical, including photocopying and recording, or by any information storage and retrieval system, without permission in writing from the copyright holder.

Views expressed in articles published are the authors', and are not to be attributed to The National Foundation or its editors unless expressly so stated.

Library of Congress Cataloging in Publication Data

Melnick, Michael.
   External ear malformations.

   (Birth defects original article series ; v. 15, no. 9)
   Bibliography: p. 129
   Includes index.
   1. Ear – Abnormalities. I. Myrianthopoulos, Ntinos Cleovoulou, joint author. II. Title. III. Series.
RG626.B63 vol. 15, no. 9 [RF187] 616'.043'08s [617.8'1]
ISBN 0-8451-1034-9   LC 79-2501

The National Foundation — March of Dimes is dedicated to the goal of preventing birth defects and ameliorating their consequences for patients, families and society.

As part of our efforts to achieve these goals, we sponsor or participate in a variety of scientific meetings where all questions relating to birth defects are freely discussed. Through our professional education program we speed the dissemination of information by publishing the proceedings of these and other meetings. From time to time, we also reprint pertinent journal articles to help achieve our goal. Now and then, in the course of these articles or discussions, individual viewpoints may be expressed which go beyond the purely scientific and into controversial matters. It should be noted, therefore, that personal viewpoints about such matters will not be censored but this does not constitute an endorsement of them by The National Foundation.

Table of Contents

Preface ix

PART I: INTRODUCTION

1. MORPHOGENESIS AND DYSMORPHOGENESIS 1
Normal Morphogenesis of the Branchial Region 1
External Ear 8
Middle Ear.. 8
Dysmorphogenesis: Concepts and Definitions...................... 11
Single Malformations and Their Possible Pathogenesis............. 11
Auricular Deformations 18
Malformation Syndromes 19

2. EPIDEMIOLOGY.. 31
The Nature of Previous Data 31
Incidence 31
Race, Ethnic and Geographic Distribution 36
Sex Distribution 37
Laterality 39
Associated Malformations 39
Syndrome Incidence 40
Summary 40

3. ETIOLOGY 41
External Ear and Branchial Cleft Malformations and
    Single Gene Mutations 41
External Ear Malformations and Chromosomal Aberrations 44
Environmental Etiologies: An Introduction........................ 45
The Placenta and Fetal Membranes 46
Infectious Agents 47
Ionizing Radiation.. 47
Pharmaceutical Preparations and Other Chemicals 48
Gene-Environment Interaction 51

PART II: MATERIALS AND METHODS

4. THE STUDY DESIGN... 55
Composition of the Present Study Population..................... 57
Data Collection 59

5. DATA ANALYSIS 61
Epidemiologic Analysis... 61
Genetic Analysis 63

viii / TABLE OF CONTENTS

PART III: RESULTS

6. GENERAL CHARACTERISTICS 69
   Etiologic Relationships 72
   Familial vs Isolated 74
   Laterality 75
   Additional Malformations in the Nonsyndromic Cases 75
   Sex Ratios 77
   Race 78
   Institution 78
   Racial and Institutional Variability 79

7. GENETICS 83
   Segregation Analysis 85
   Parental Age, Mutation and the Sporadic Cases 91

8. ENVIRONMENTAL VARIABLES 95
   The Hemorrhage Hypothesis 96
   Birth Order 99
   Socioeconomic Status 100
   Chronic Diseases During Pregnancy 101
   Infectious Diseases During the First Trimester 101
   Maternal Vaccinations During the First Trimester 102
   Other Complications of Pregnancy 103
   Drug Use During the First Trimester 103
   Gene–Environment Interaction: Twins 104

9. NATURAL HISTORY 107
   Birthweight and Isolated External Ear Malformations 107
   Intelligence (IQ) 108
   Hearing 110
   Speech Production 114

PART IV: DISCUSSION AND SUMMARY

10. DISCUSSION 117
    Racial Variability 117
    Genetic Considerations 118
    Genetic Counseling 119
    Environmental Considerations 120
    Syndrome Identification 120
    Classification of External Ear and/or Branchial Cleft
      Malformations 122
    Natural History 124

11. SUMMARY 127

References 129
Index 137

Preface

In this treatise we seek to investigate what mankind perceives as an abnormal ear, not necessarily in function but in design. How do we judge an ear to be abnormal? Need we catalog and measure its component parts and compare them to thousands of such previous observations? Hardly! Man perceives his fellow man as a broad impression of geometric shapes and the "gestalt" derived from the interrelation of these shapes defines for him, in a very biased way, normality. Our definition of a normal ear is, in our daily lives, not the one outlined in "Gray's Anatomy." Instead it is the one provided by Kimon Nicolaides, one of America's greatest teachers of drawing: "The ear fundamentally is a little funnel. Do not think of it, as many people do, as a kind of design stuck on the side of the head. Keep in mind the fact that all the little lines and forms are made to catch the sound and carry it around so that it enters the hole of the ear. All the channels lead into the funnel." Those ears which do not satisfy this perception constitute a flaw in Nature's invention and provide the raison d'etre for the efforts to follow.

Removing the panache, it can be stated in a more mundane way that the specific aim of this investigation was to identify the epidemiologic, genetic and possible environmental parameters characteristic of malformations of the external ear. Further, it was the aim of the study to assess the clinical significance of these malformations with regard to hearing loss, IQ, renal malfunction, and other relevant variables.

This is publication number 78-23 from the Department of Medical Genetics and was supported in part by the Indiana University Human Genetics Center Grant PHS GM 21054 and NIH Postdoctoral Individual Fellowship Award DE 01274.

We wish to acknowledge the generous advice of Dr. David Bixler (syndromology), Dr. P. Michael Conneally (segregation analysis), Dr. Pao-Lo Yu (statistics), and Dr. Kenneth S. Brown (embryology) during the data analysis and critical reading of this manuscript. A special thanks is due Dr. Walter E. Nance for his characteristically diligent and perceptive advice and criticism throughout the execution of this project.

Finally, the study and present report would not have been possible without the support and generosity of Dr. A. Donald Merritt, the untiring administrative assistance of Ms. Kristan Lucas and secretarial assistance of Mrs. Lisa Gabrielsen, and most of all the continued tolerance by Anita, Cliff and Lynn of one man's (M.M.) never ending peregrination.

Michael Melnick, DDS, PhD

PART I
INTRODUCTION

1. Morphogenesis and Dysmorphogenesis

NORMAL MORPHOGENESIS
OF THE BRANCHIAL REGION

Although it is not the purpose of this report to provide a detailed discussion of the branchial region and its development, any study that concerns itself with dysmorphology demands at the outset a working knowledge of normal morphogenesis. The discussion that follows is but a brief synopsis. The reader is referred to Moore (1973), Tuchmann-Duplessis et al (1972), Tuchmann-Duplessis and Haegel (1974), Tuchmann-Duplessis et al (1974), Corliss (1976), Rogers (1968) and Anson and Donaldson (1973) for a more complete description.

The formation of the head and neck is intimately associated with the fate of the branchial apparatus. In the lateral endodermal walls of the anterior part of the foregut there are formed five *pharyngeal pouches,* the first four of which extend outward to meet the corresponding ectodermal grooves or *branchial clefts.* On either side of the branchial clefts lie rounded swellings which are termed *branchial arches.* The arches thicken by mesenchymal cell migration, division, and condensation leaving the thin, primarily ectodermal-endodermal, *branchial closing membranes* between them. These membranes, then, represent a rather precarious separation between the foregut and the external environment of the embryo.

This whole process begins around the 20th day of embryonic life and by the 28th day four well-developed pairs of branchial arches are visible (Fig. 1-1). The 5th and 6th branchial arches are rudimentary in man but their corresponding aortic arches do arise, the 6th more evident than the transitory 5th (Tuchmann-Duplessis and Haegel, 1974). Each arch at day-28 typically contains an aortic arch artery, a cartilaginous bar and a muscle component, as well as a nerve.

At about day-30 there is a rapid growth of the 2nd branchial arch over the 3rd and 4th arches and 2nd, 3rd and 4th clefts to form a single ectodermal depression known as the cervical sinus (Fig. 1-2). The 2nd arch eventually fuses with the ectoderm in an area corresponding to the 6th arch and by day-48 the 2nd, 3rd and 4th

2 / INTRODUCTION

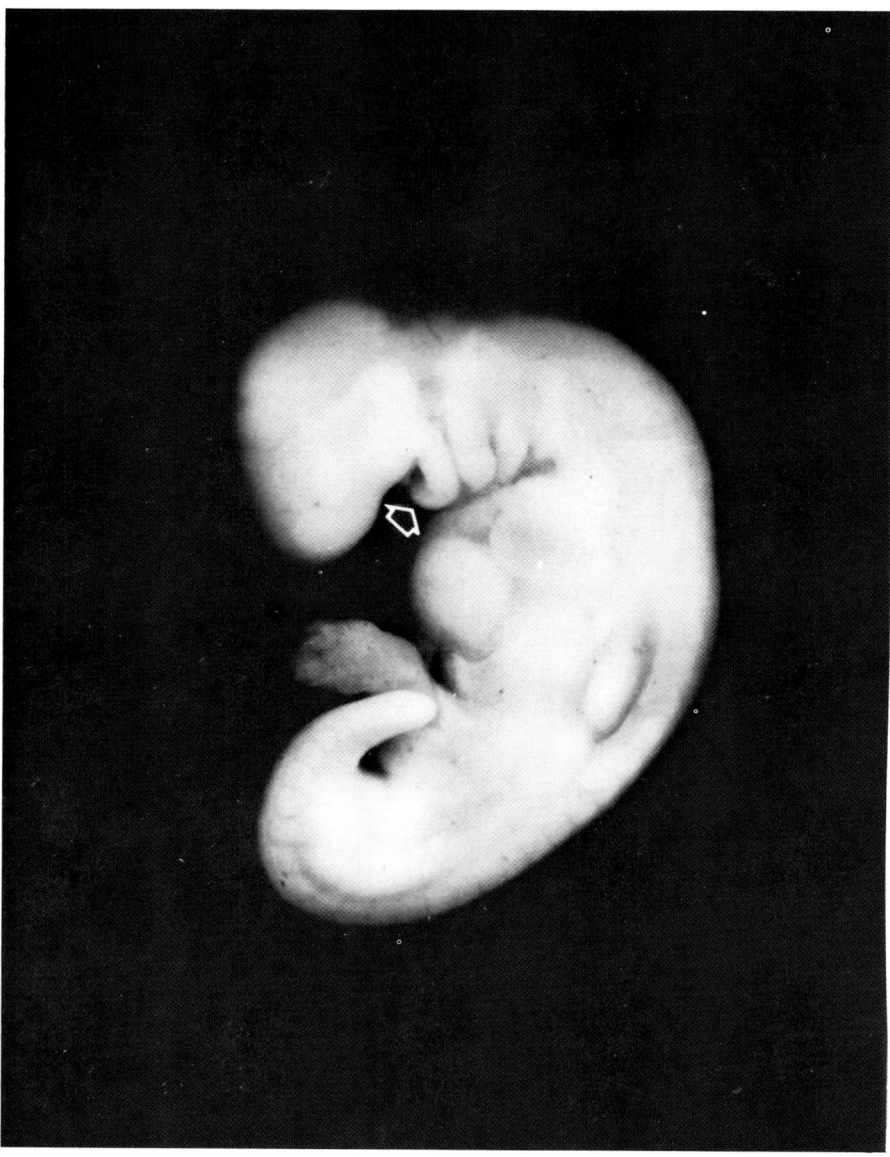

Fig. 1-1. Lateral view of human embryo at Carnegie stage 13 (length: 4-6 mm; age: circa 28 days). Note the presence of 4 well-defined branchial arches (arrow), designated from left to right as I (mandibular arch), II (hyoid arch), III, and IV. (Figs. 1-1 – 1-5 Courtesy of Professor Hideo Nishimura, Central Institute for Experimental Animals, Kawasaki, Japan).

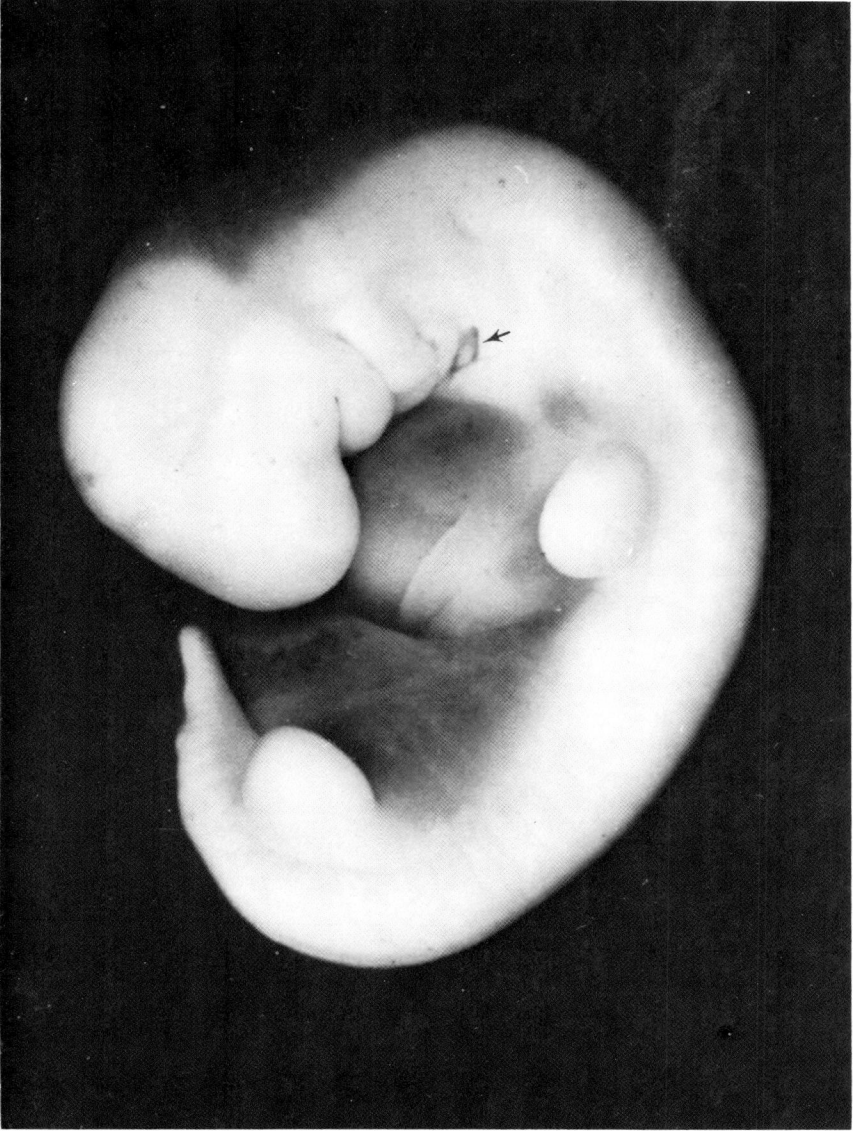

Fig. 1-2. Lateral view of human embryo at Carnegie stage 14 (length: 5-7 mm; age: circa 32 days). Note that branchial arch II grows over arches III and IV and the corresponding clefts, eventually resulting in only a single ectodermal depression termed the cervical sinus (arrow).

4 / INTRODUCTION

arches are obliterated along with the cervical sinus to give a smooth contour to the neck (Fig. 1-3). Only the dorsal end of the first branchial cleft remains (Fig. 1-4) to form the epithelium of the external auditory meatus. By this time the auricular hillocks or swellings arising from the 1st and 2nd arches have fused as part of the ongoing process of external ear formation (Fig. 1-5).

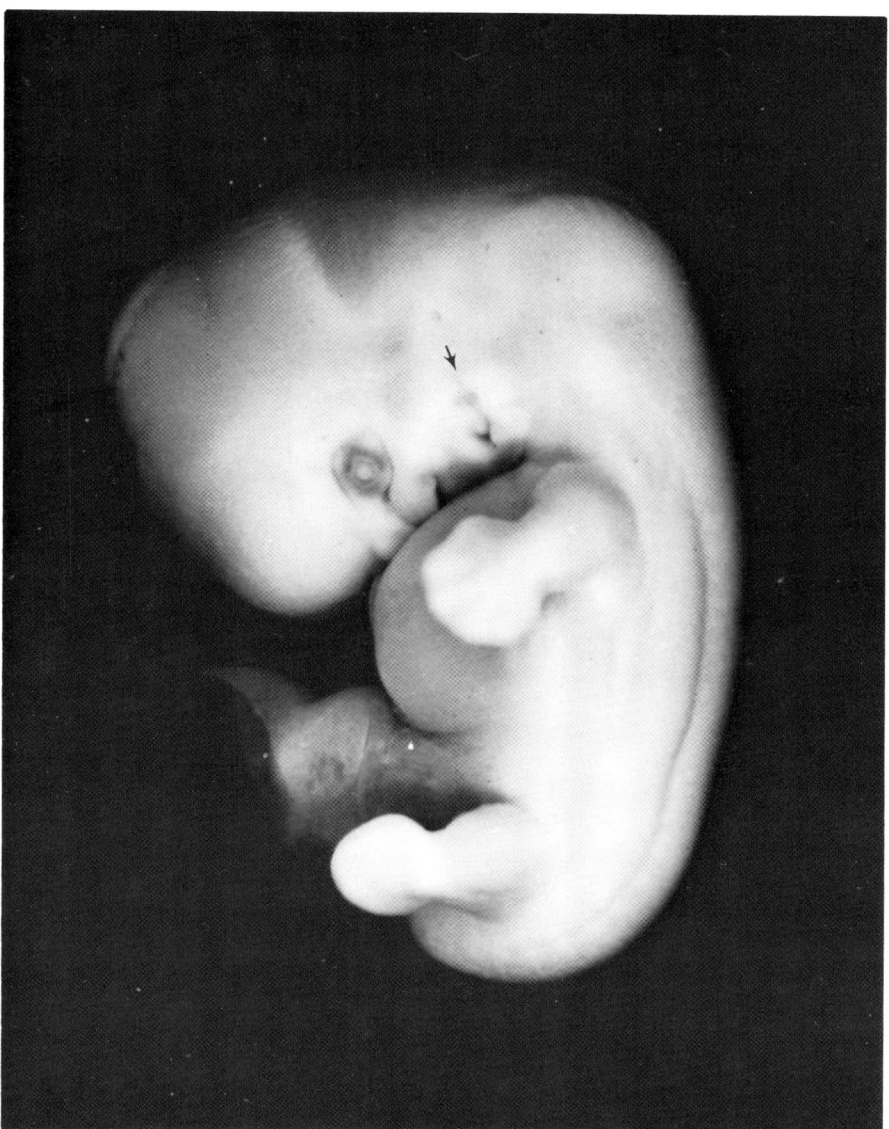

Fig. 1-3. Lateral view of human embryo at Carnegie stage 18 (length: 13-17 mm; age: circa 44 days). The arrow points to the 6 auricular hillocks which have begun to fuse around the 1st branchial cleft; the cervical sinus is no longer present.

Morphogenesis and Dysmorphogenesis / 5

It should be noted here that there is now substantial evidence that neural crest cells in large numbers migrate around the head to reinforce the developing branchial arch structures (Johnston 1975; LeDouarin, 1975; Noden, 1975). The neural crest is initially composed of ectodermal cells found at the junction between neural plate and surface ectoderm. In the head region nearly all the crest cells migrate be-

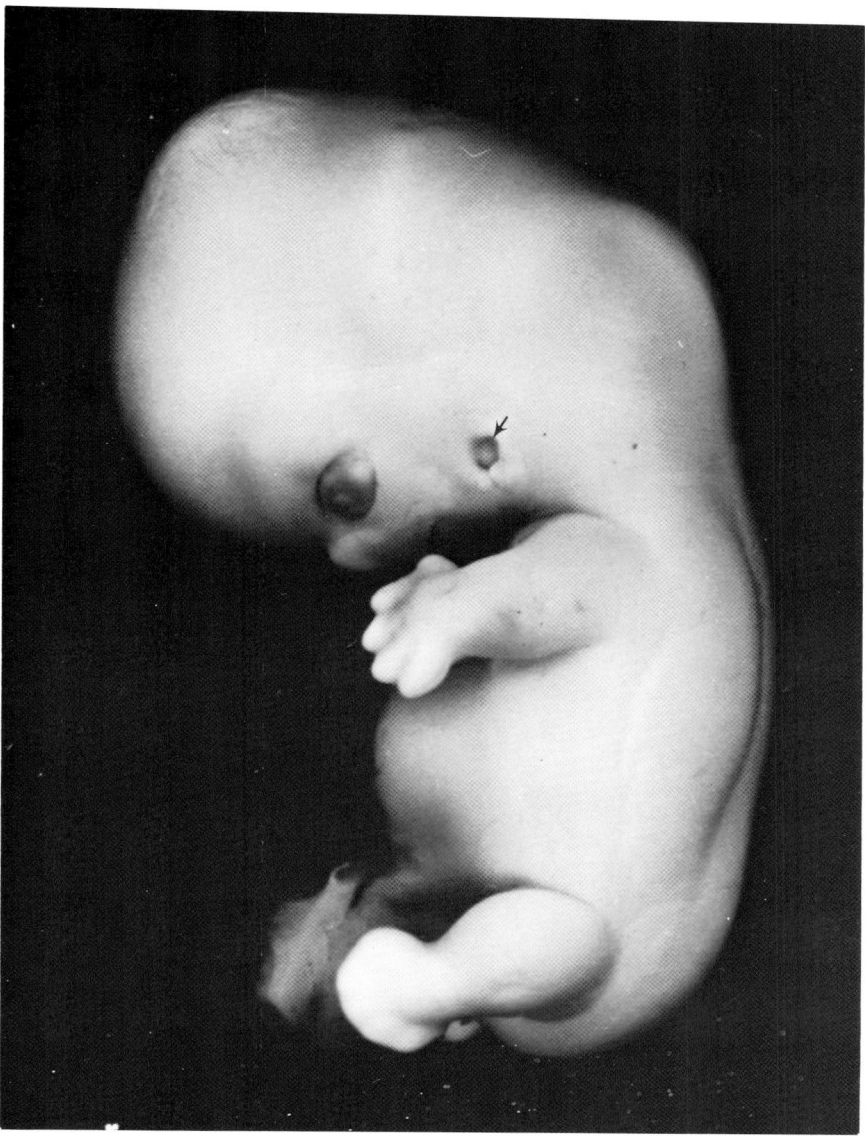

Fig. 1-4. Lateral view of human embryo at Carnegie stage 19 (length: 16-18 mm; age: circa 47.5 days). Note that the auricular hillocks have completely fused and the external auditory meatus (arrow) is now well-defined.

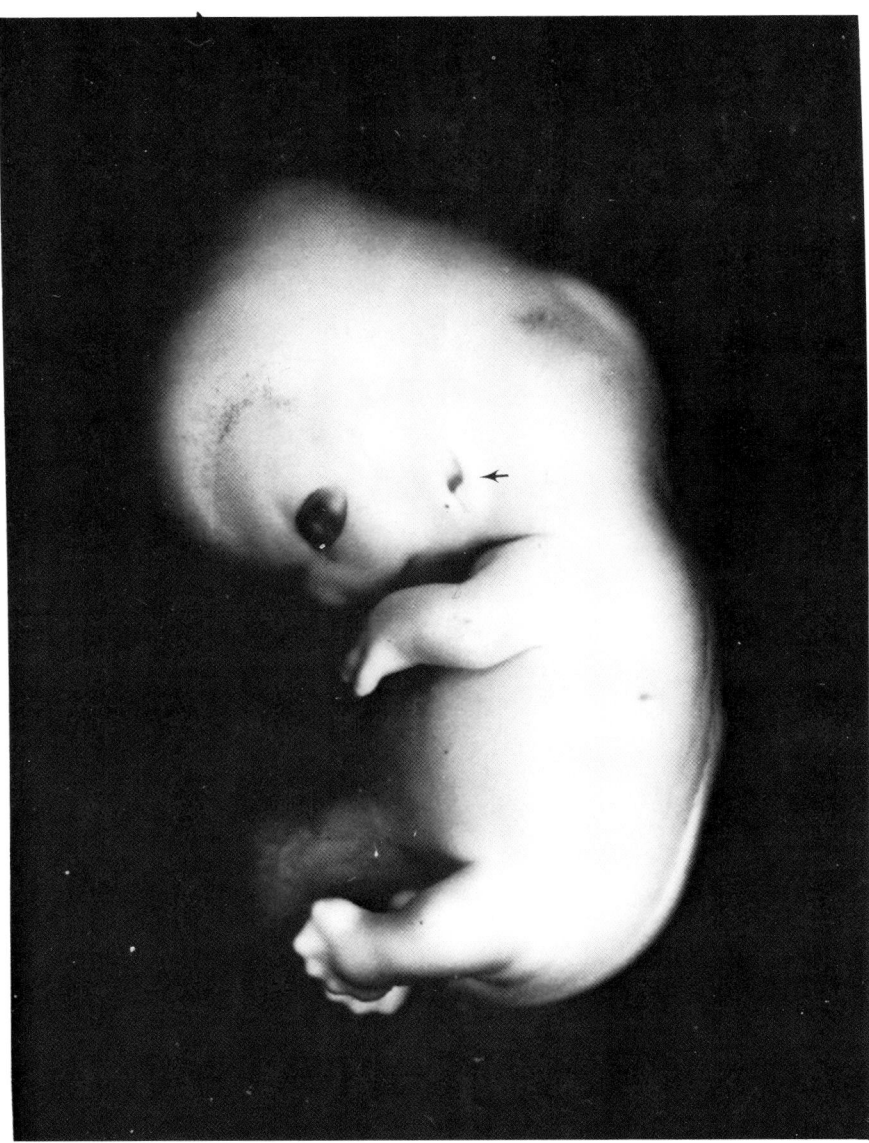

Fig. 1-5. Lateral view of human embryo at Carnegie stage 20 (length: 18-22 mm; age: circa 50.5 days). Note that the fused hillocks have continued to differentiate into a recognizable rudimentary pinna (arrow).

tween this surface ectoderm and the existing mesoderm. Since neural crest cells proliferate actively, they become the main cellular component of the branchial arches (Le Douarin, 1975). This relationship is pictured in Figure 1-6. The derivatives of this migrating neural crest are numerous including both the mandibular (1st) and hyoid (2nd) arch cartilages. In fact, the only major components of the face not of crest origin are the retina and lens, epithelial tissues, vascular endothelia and most skeletal muscle.

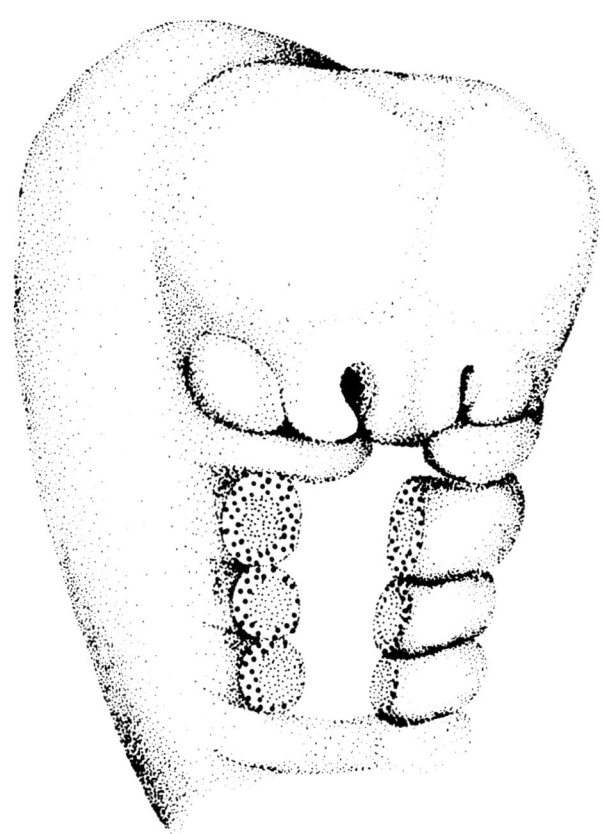

Fig. 1-6. Schematic diagram of a vertebrate embryo showing the relation between neural crest (heavy stipple) and mesoderm (light stipple) in developing branchial arches. Skeletal and connective tissues develop from the crest component, while endothelial and voluntary skeletal muscle cells form from the mesodermal cores. (From Johnston MC: The neural crest in abnormalities of the face and brain. Birth defects 11(7):1-18, 1975. With permission.)

EXTERNAL EAR

The external ear is derived from the ectoderm and mesenchyme of the 1st and 2nd branchial arches. At about day-38 the smooth margins of the 1st and 2nd arches begin to develop small tubercules or *hillocks*. Three such hillocks appear on the caudal border of the mandibular arch and three on the cephalic border of the second arch (Fig. 1-3). These swellings are the result of mesenchymal proliferation. By day 41 the hillocks have reached their maximum size, have moved in a more dorsal and lateral direction and have begun to fuse. This fusion is complete by the 43rd–45th day of embryonic life (Figs. 1-4 and 1-5). At about this time the amount of mesenchyme in the 1st and 2nd arches is about equal. However from about the end of the 7th week or the beginning of the 8th through subsequent fetal development the amount of hyoid arch mesenchyme increases substantially relative to the mandibular arch mesenchyme. By the 20th week of development the ear is nearly anatomically complete. The only portions of the ear derived from the 1st arch are the tragus and possibly the anterior crus of the helix margin while the 2nd arch derivatives include the helix, anthelix, scapha, antitragus and the lobule (Fig. 1-7). Finally, it should be noted that the auricles begin their development in a region roughly corresponding to the upper part of the future neck and as the mandible develops they move in a dorsolateral direction to take their normal position lateral to and at the level of the eye.

The dorsal end of the 1st branchial cleft is beginning to widen while the auricle is developing and by day-41 it becomes a distinct structure termed the *fossa angularis*. The ectodermal cells at the bottom of this fossa proliferate and extend inward as a solid core known as the *meatal plug* (Fig. 1-8). By the 70th day of development this plug begins to approach the expanding tympanic cavity and its central cells are degenerating to form a cavity which ultimately becomes the *external auditory meatus* (Fig. 1-8).

MIDDLE EAR

The middle ear is derived from the *tubotympanic recess* of the 1st pharyngeal pouch which eventually gives rise to the epithelia of the eustachian tube and tympanic cavity as well as the mastoid cavities (Fig. 1-8). The distal end of the 1st pouch grows in the direction of the external auditory meatus to form the tympanic cavity and the proximal end becomes the eustachian tube. As the tympanic cavity expands it gradually envelops the middle ear ossicles, their tendons and ligaments and the chorda tympani nerve. By the end of the 6th month, the distal wall of the tympanic cavity approximates the proximal end of the external auditory meatus. This results in a trilayer of ectodermal and endodermal epithelium separated by a thin fibrous layer, altogether termed the *tympanic membrane* (Anson and Donaldson, 1973).

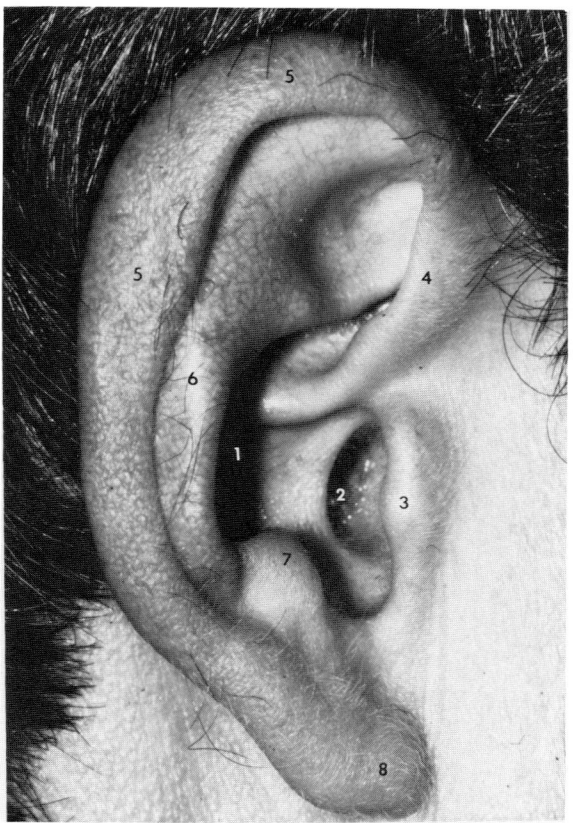

Fig. 1-7. "Normal" external ear: 1) concha; 2) external auditory meatus; 3) tragus; 4) crus helix; 5) helix; 6) anthelix; 7) antitragus; 8) lobule.

During the 2nd month the ossicles differentiate from the mesenchyme surrounding the tubotympanic recess (Fig. 1-8). First the Reichert cartilage (2nd arch) gives rise to the *stapes* and then the dorsal end of the Meckel cartilage (1st arch) gives rise to the *incus* and *malleus*. The stapes first appears as a ring encircling a small vessel, the stapedial artery, which subsequently undergoes atrophy. The stapes originally is continuous with the otic capsular area around its foot-plate (Hough, 1963). This otic capsular area begins to thin out and the cells develop into fibrous tissue and not precartilage. That portion of the otic capsule opposite the footplate of the stapes remains very thin to eventually give rise to the *fenestra vestibuli* or oval window which transmits sound vibrations to the inner ear. The footplate's circumference is covered with hyaline cartilage and is attached to the margin of the

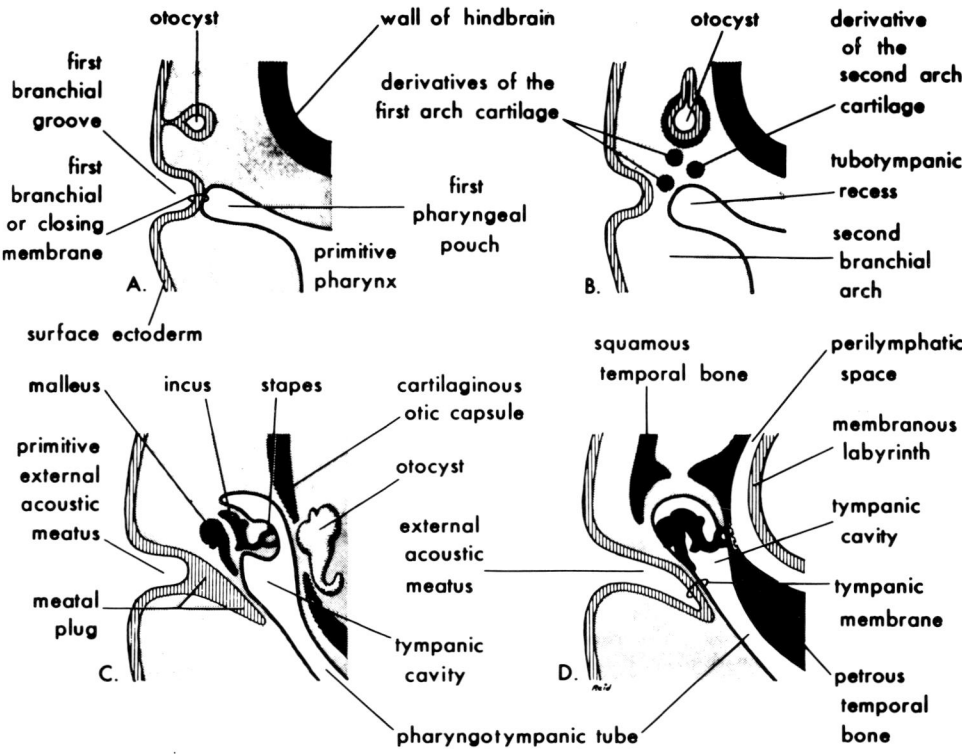

Fig. 1-8. Schematic representation of the developing middle ear: A) circa 4 weeks—note the relation of the otocyst (inner ear primordia) to the branchial apparatus; B) circa 5 weeks—note the tubotympanic recess (future tympanic cavity) and branchial arch cartilages; C) later stage—the tubotympanic recess has begun to envelop the ossicles; D) final stage—note the relation of the middle ear to the inner ear (perilymphatic space, membranous labyrinth, etc) and the external auditory (acoustic) meatus. (From Moore KL: *The Developing Human, Clinically Oriented Embryology*. 2nd Ed. Philadelphia: WB Saunders Company, 1977. With permission.)

fenestra vestibuli by a fibrous ring, the *annular ligament*. The tympanic cavity ultimately contains a chain of three movable ossicles (Fig. 1-8), the malleus attached to the tympanic membrane, the stapes to the outer rim of the oval window and the incus placed between and connected to the malleus by a diarthroidal joint and to the stapes by an enarthroidal joint. When, after birth, the tympanic cavity then fills with air (via the eustachian tube) the middle ear system is fully set to transmit vibrations to the inner ear for neurologic processing.

DYSMORPHOGENESIS: CONCEPTS AND DEFINITIONS

Congenital malformations are structural abnormalities at birth which result from untoward events during the *critical periods* of embryogenesis, generally between the 3rd to 12th week of postconceptional age in humans (Nishimura and Tanimura, 1976). The critical period, then, is the entire period during which a given malformation can be induced. Each organ system is thought to have its own unique critical period(s) during which dysmorphogenesis may be initiated. For the ear this is from the 4th to 12th week, postconception. It should be remembered, however, that some development continues until late gestation or sometime during early postnatal life and the presence of teratogens subsequent to the so-called critical period may also interfere with cell proliferation, cell differentiation and/or cell migration. The end result would most likely not be gross dysmorphology, but microscopic hypoplasias, dysplasias and heterotopias. Although most studies involve those malformations which present themselves at the gross or macroscopic level, this represents methodologic convenience and not necessarily accuracy. There is no a priori reason to exclude the possibility that microscopic malformations can indeed be associated with postnatal dysfunction simply because they may be difficult to detect.

When one reads the literature of dysmorphology, one quickly discovers the terms *agenesis, hypoplasia, dysplasia* and *heterotopia*. As used in this report, *agenesis (aplasia)* is the total absence of an organ or body part, *hypoplasia* is an underdevelopment characterized by small size with normal gross and histologic morphology, *dysplasia* refers to gross and/or histologic disorganization or atypical differentiation of a particular tissue or organ system, including congenital neoplasms, hamartomas and metaplasias, and *heterotopia* refers to the presence of tissue in an abnormal location. Two other terms that should be defined are *hyperplasia,* an increase in the number of normal cells in normal arrangement in a tissue, and *hypertrophy,* the enlargement of an organ or body part due to an increase in the size of its constituent cells. Finally, when there is doubt about the particular pathologic nature of the defect, the terms dysmorphic or dysmorphia are used.

The specific developmental phenomena preceding the dysmorphic states just mentioned can broadly be classified as abnormal cell migration or movement, abnormal cell proliferation and atypical cell death (Johnston and Pratt, 1975). These phenomena are not mutually exclusive. For example, a mass of cells may migrate late or not at all and thus miss the chance for a specifically timed inductive interaction with its normally juxtaposed partner. Another example might be the case of abnormal differentiation leading to a failure of programmed cell death and thus a failure of a structure to canalize.

SINGLE MALFORMATIONS AND THEIR POSSIBLE PATHOGENESIS

The pathogenesis of most human congenital malformations is not known, includ-

12 / INTRODUCTION

ing that of the external ear. Nevertheless, reasonable deductions from animal models may be appropriate and what follows is a discussion of various malformations of the external and middle ear and their likely pathogenesis.

External Ear:

   a) *Anotia* (agenesis of the auricle) denotes complete absence of the external ear. This malformation probably results from failure of the auricular hillocks to develop through mesenchymal proliferation.

   b) *Microtia* (Fig. 1-9) is a severely disorganized (dysplastic) external ear usually found as rudimentary structures resembling a malformed lobule or a series of remnants similar in anatomy to that seen in the 6th week of embryonic life. The origin

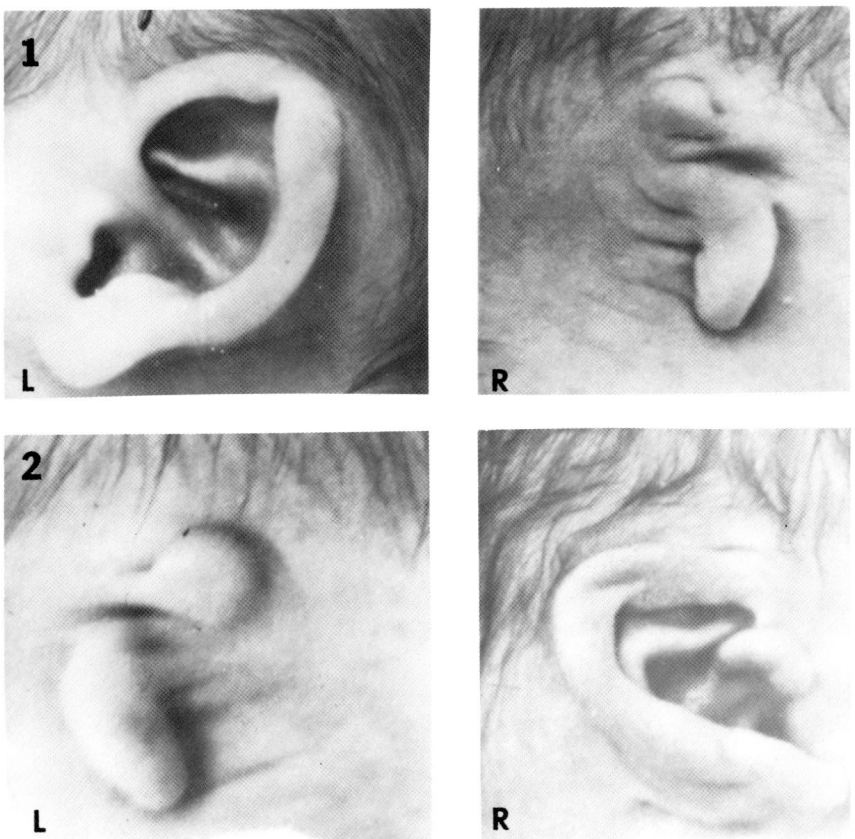

Fig. 1-9. Microtia in a pair of monozygotic twins. Note that the right ear of Twin 1 is severely microtic and the left ear is relatively normal, while the left ear of Twin 2 is severely microtic and the right ear is mildly microtic. (From Holmes LB: *Common Birth Defects: The Normal and Malformed Newborn*. Boston: Embryology Press, 1979. With permission.)

of this anomaly appears to be a decreased proliferation of the auricular hillocks and/or a defect in the fusion of these hillocks. Atresia of the external auditory meatus and middle ear anomalies frequently accompany the microtia, resulting in conductive hearing loss. In 1972 Harada and Ishii reported on clinical and anatomic studies in 57 patients with congenital microtia. During middle ear surgery the auditory ossicles were evaluated as to the extent of dysmorphia. In general, increasing severity of unilateral microtia was associated with increasing ossicular malformations. However, if one looks at their data more carefully, it is interesting to note that bilateral cases were often asymmetric and the severity of the ossicular malformations had an inverse relationship to the severity of microtia.

c) *Lop ears* are a downward folding and/or deficiency of the helix and scapha in association with inadequate development of the anthelix while *cup ears* (Fig. 1-10), having many of these same features, protrude because of the excessively concave concha (Rogers, 1968). *Protruding ears* have a normal vertical height with a poorly formed anthelix, excessive conchal cartilage, an increased angle of protrusion of the lobule and an inadequate folding of the helix margin (Rogers, 1968). All three types of malformations probably represent varying degrees of faulty differentiation (dysplasia) of the 2nd branchial arch hillocks, but to a degree considerably less than microtia. Jaffe (1976) has documented the occurrence of ossicular malforma-

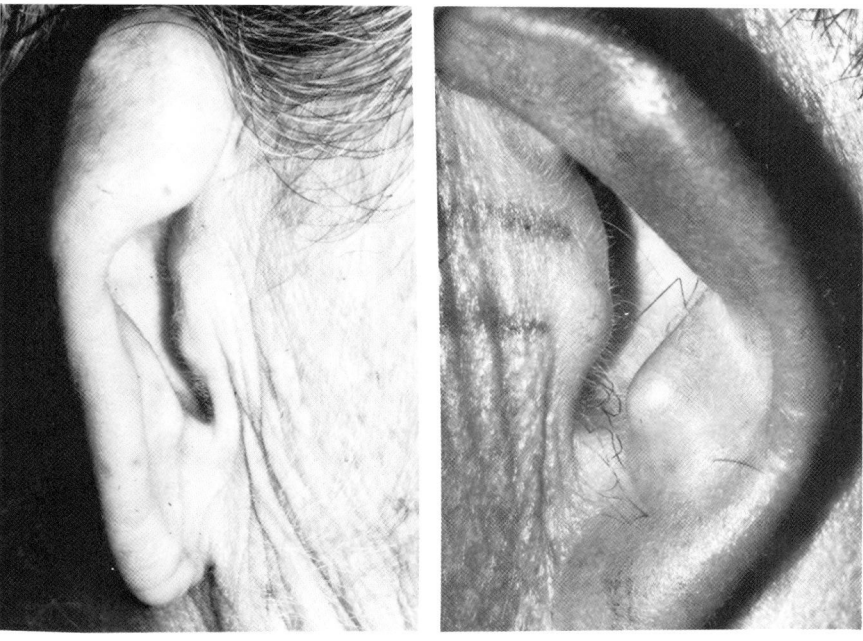

Fig. 1-10. Note the lopping and cupping of the external ears of these 2 patients with severe conductive hearing loss.

14 / INTRODUCTION

tions in nonsyndromic cases of these ear anomalies but as yet the frequency of middle ear anomalies with these types of pinna malformations is unknown.

d) *Anomalies of the lobule* are rare and usually take the form of complete absence (agenesis) or a lobule coloboma. They both may result from a failure of the most caudal 2nd arch hillock to develop completely but in varying degrees.

e) *Cryptotia,* a very rare anomaly, is an abnormal adherence of the helix and anthelix to the head. Since the upper part of the auricle becomes detached from the head in the 4th month of gestation, cryptotia is attributed to persistence of this fetal attachment (Warkany, 1971). This malformation, then, is probably associated with a failure of programmed cell death or secondary reattachment.

f) *Atresia of the external auditory meatus* is of two types, osseous or membranous, and is usually associated with varying severities of microtia. This malformation results from a failure of the meatal plug to canalize, another aural dysplasia likely to be related to a failure of programmed cell death.

g) *Auricular sinuses and fistulas* are usually preauricular and are most often located at the anterior margin of the ascending limb of the helix (Fig. 1-11). Other preauricular fistulas and sinuses can occasionally be found along a hyperbolic curve which separates the tragus from the remaining pinna and extends from the temple to that part of the cheek adjacent to the ear (Black et al, 1973). It has generally been accepted that the preauricular fistulas and sinuses represent incomplete

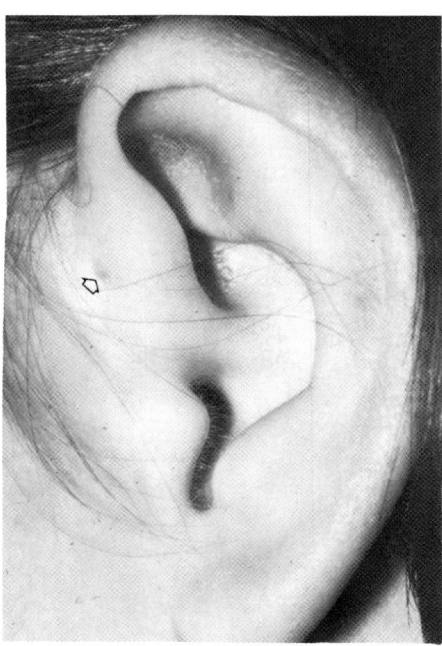

Fig. 1-11. Preauricular pit (arrow) in its most frequently found position, prehelical.

fusion of the 1st arch hillocks. However, since they are not necessarily at points of fusion, this is not a completely satisfactory explanation. Some have suggested that they may be related to defective closure of the most dorsal part of the 1st branchial cleft (Moore, 1973), while others say they represent ectodermal folds that are sequestered during auricle formation (Aronsohn et al, 1976). More rarely a sinus can be found in the center of the lobule. This may represent the mildest expression of the lobule dysplasia discussed above.

h) *Auricular appendages* (tags) are also usually preauricular (Fig. 1-12) but on occasion can be found within the ear, behind the ear or on the lobule. The most frequent location of these tags is pretragal but they can be found anywhere along the hyperbolic curve described above, or along a line extending from the tragus to the angle of the mouth. Rarely, they may be found as far down as the sternoclavicular area. These tags vary in size, may be sessile or pedunculated, and are composed of skin and sometimes cartilage. They may or may not be associated with other auricular abnormalities. Occasionally they are so well developed that they simulate an extra pinna which has resulted in the misnomer "accessory auricle." These appendages are thought to result from the development of accessory auricular hillocks (Moore, 1973) perhaps because of ectopic migration and/or induction.

i) *Macrotia* is an ear with normal architecture but larger than normal size. This anomaly probably represents a true hyperplasia and presumably would be due to

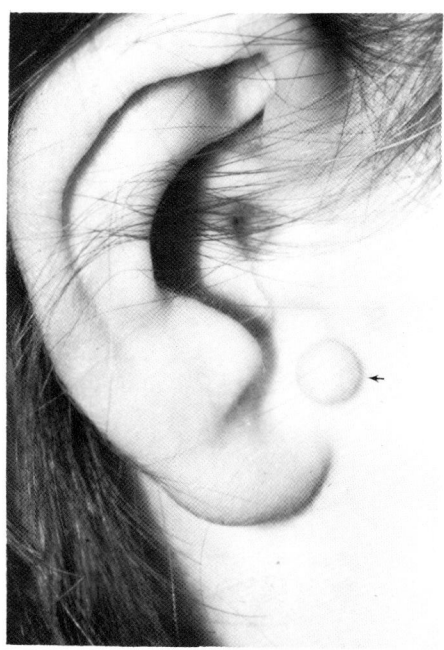

Fig. 1-12. Preauricular tag (arrow).

excessive mesenchymal proliferation in the 6 auricular hillocks.

j) *Micro-ear* is an ear with normal architecture but smaller than normal size. The terminology is unfortunate but the alternative, microtia, has been used for so many years to describe small, *dysplastic* ears that it is not really applicable here. This anomaly is probably representative of a true hypoplasia and presumably would be due to deficient mesenchymal proliferation in all 6 auricular hillocks or subsequent growth failure after full, normal formation. The determination of micro-ear and macrotia ("macro-ear") may be made by using the standards in Figure 1-13.

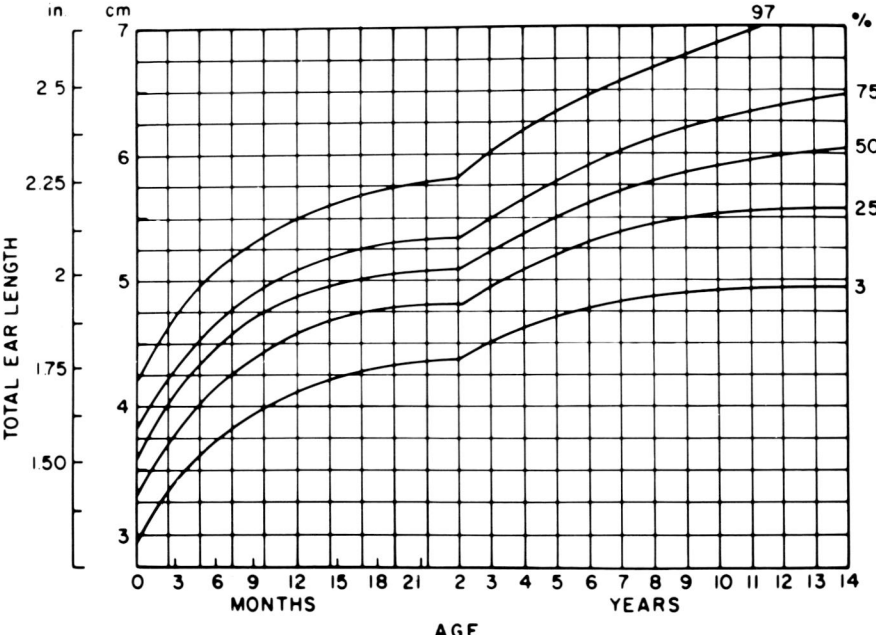

Fig. 1-13. Total ear length by age. Length obtained by measuring the distance between the most inferior and superior portions of the ear; sex correction — add 1.5 mm to measured length for females and subtract 1.5 mm from measured length for males. (From Feingold M, Bossert WH: Normal values for selected physical parameters: An aid to syndrome delineation. Birth Defects 10(13):11, 1974. With permission.)

Middle Ear:

a) *Tympanic cavity anomalies* are of two types, narrowing or absence. In both cases one can find cavity space replaced by spongy bone (Warkany, 1971). Depending on the severity of closure and ossicular malformation, there will be varying degrees of conductive deafness. Since the tympanic cavity arises from the already present distal end of the 1st pharyngeal pouch, the nature of the pathogenesis of this dysplasia remains unclear.

b) *Congenital fixation of the stapes* is not uncommon and results in severe conductive deafness. This malformation may exist in the presence or absence of other external and/or middle ear abnormalities. Failure of differentiation (dysplasia) of the fibrous annular ligament attached to the footplate of the stapes results in fixation of the stapes to the otic capsule by ossification (Moore, 1973).

c) *Persistent stapedial artery* is occasionally found during exploratory tympanotomy and may represent another failure of programmed cell death of a transitory fetal structure or a compensatory persistence for a hydrodynamically inadequate "replacement" vasculature.

d) *Malformations of the incus and malleus* are most often expressed as incomplete or atypical differentiation of the dorsal end of the Meckel cartilage. This dysplasia is seen as either malformed individual ossicles or a bony union of the two bones with varying degrees of architectural similarity to their normal counterparts.

e) *Malformations of the eustachian tube* are not common but absence of the tube, atresia of the lumen, atresia of the ostium pharyngium and angular bends have been described (Warkany, 1971). This agenesis or dysplasia is due to faulty differentiation of the proximal end of the 1st pharyngeal pouch.

Branchial Cleft and/or Pouch Anomalies

These anomalies are of 4 types, primarily, *external branchial sinuses, internal branchial sinuses, communicating branchial fistulas* and *lateral cervical cysts.* The sinuses and fistulas are lined with epithelium and occasionally vestigial remnants of the branchial arch cartilages may be present. External branchial sinuses represent incomplete obliteration of the branchial clefts; internal branchial sinuses represent incomplete obliteration of the pharyngeal pouch; communicating branchial fistulas represent both an external and internal pair of branchial sinuses which communicate because of a perforation of the characteristically unreinforced branchial closing membranes. It seems likely that these anomalies come about by either a failure of programmed cell death of these transitory fetal structures and/or a failure of the branchial arch mesoderm to migrate into these fissures in sufficient quantity.

Sinuses that open below the angle of the mandible and course to the cartilage of the external ear are considered to be remnants of the 1st branchial cleft (Whitson, 1968). Aronsohn et al (1976) state that there are two distinct anomalies of the 1st branchial cleft. Type I is ectodermal and is a lesion of the 1st cleft only. The primary cystic mass may be anterior and inferior to the lobule and associated with the parotid gland. Drainage may occur anywhere along the lesion. Type II is ectodermal and mesodermal and has contributions from the 1st branchial cleft and also from portions of the 1st and 2nd branchial arches. This type may have openings in the upper part of the neck or external auditory canal or both. Both types are considered as duplication anomalies of either the membranous (type I) or membranous and cartilaginous (type II) portions of the external auditory canal. It should be noted that neither type is associated with pretragal cysts or sinuses.

Those sinuses that pass between the internal and external carotid arteries are remnants of the 2nd branchial cleft, and those sinuses that are lateral to both vessels are remnants of the 3rd branchial cleft (Proctor and Proctor, 1970). Nearly all of the reported branchial sinus anomalies arise from the 2nd branchial cleft and/or pouch. They exit inferior to the hyoid and anterior to the sternocleidomastoid muscle (Fig. 1-14).

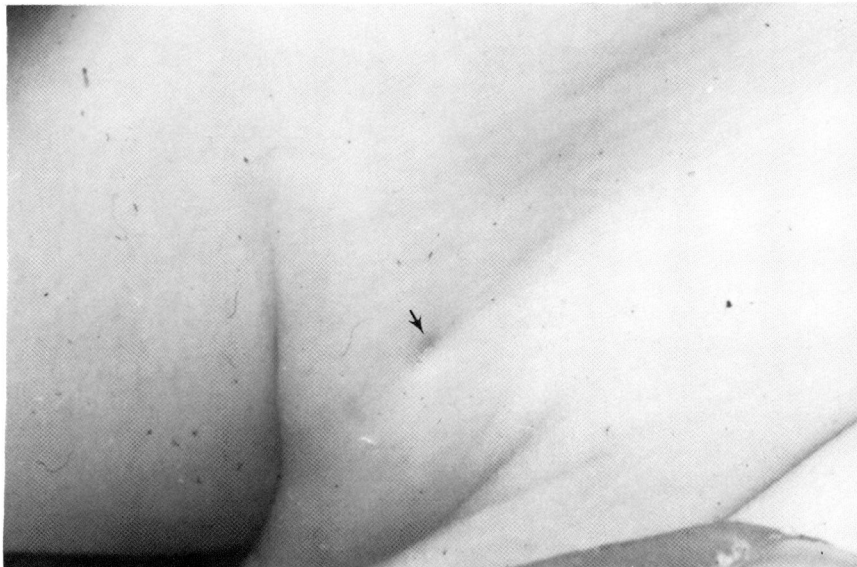

Fig. 1-14. Branchial cleft sinus (arrow) in an infant.

Lateral cervical cysts are found at the level of the hyoid bone and anterior to the sternocleidomastoid. Since they characteristically have abundant lymphoreticular tissue with germinal centers, they are thought to arise from epithelial inclusions in lymph nodes during the time of cervical sinus obliteration (Bhaskar and Bernier, 1959). These are true inclusion cysts and should be distinguished from 2nd branchial cleft and/or pouch sinuses and fistulas.

AURICULAR DEFORMATIONS

In recent years much attention has been given to maldevelopment that may arise in the fetus when the amniotic fluid volume falls to a level which no longer permits free fetal movements. As the placenta ages, there is occasionally premature continuous leakage from partially ruptured membranes. Fetal oliguria or anuria secondary to renal malformation may also give rise to a decreased amniotic fluid volume. Regardless of the antecedent event, oligohydramnios is frequently associated with congenital *deformations* as distinguished from malformations. Deformations characteristically arise late in fetal life and can be seen as postural or plastic alterations of morphology of a previously normally formed structure. Although there is a 2% incidence of such deformations, 90% of these will correct spontaneously after birth and nearly all of the remaining 10% will do so with early postural assistance (Dunn, 1976).

Since the entire fetus benefits from the protection offered by amniotic fluid against the pressure of the uterus, all parts of the unborn child may be affected by oligohydramniotic postural molding mechanisms. Of particular interest here is the so-called Potter syndrome consisting of pulmonary hypoplasia, abnormal limb positioning and "compression facies," including large, flattened auricles. The primary defect is oligohydramnios which may result from bilateral renal agenesis or severe dysplasia or from other causes of decreased amniotic fluid (Barr and Burdi, 1976). Dunn (1976) presents evidence that all types of deformations share several pregnancy characteristics, including primigravidity, maternal hypertension, breech presentation and fetal growth retardation. Nevertheless, both human (Dunn, 1976) and animal (Poswillo, 1966) data strongly implicate oligohydramnios as the "kingpost" in the causal chain of postural fetal deformation.

MALFORMATION SYNDROMES

The primary external ear malformation syndromes may be thought of in 4 groups: otomandibular, branchio-oto-dysplasia, ear dysplasia-renal adysplasia, and variable system. There are many malformation syndromes, genetic and nongenetic, which have ear malformations but those to be described below constitute syndromes in which the dysmorphic ear is an outstanding feature. The decision as to what is "outstanding" is, to be sure, highly subjective.

The otomandibular group includes the so-called "first and second branchial arch syndrome" (oculoauriculovertebral dysplasia, hemifacial microsomia), mandibulofacial dysostosis (Treacher Collins syndrome), and the otomandibular dysostosis of Konigsmark and Gorlin. Perhaps the least biased tabulation of the phenotypic expression of the *first and second branchial arch (FSBA) syndrome* (Fig. 1-15) is that of Grabb (1965). In its fullest expression, a patient with this syndrome would present with unilateral or occasionally bilateral but asymmetric underdevelopment of the external ear, middle ear, mandible, zygoma, maxilla, temporal bone, facial muscles, muscles of mastication, palatal muscles, tongue and parotid gland, as well as macrostomia, a first branchial cleft sinus, and varying degrees of facial nerve paresis. The external ear malformations include microtia, preauricular tags and/or quently cleft palate. About 75% of the patients have a lower eyelid coloboma (Gorlin et al, 1976). The pinnae are usually malformed, including microtia, hypoplasia, cupping, preauricular tags, and preauricular sinuses. The middle ear ossicles are often malformed including fusion of the malleus and incus and fixation of the stapes footplate. This syndrome is characteristically bilateral and the malformations are usually symmetric (Fig. 1-16). However, the expression is highly variable and the family members should be examined carefully for minor expression of the syndrome before declaring a sporadic case a new mutation.

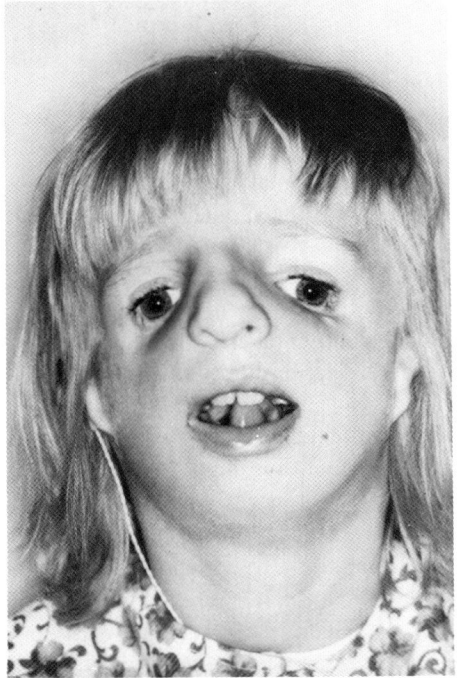
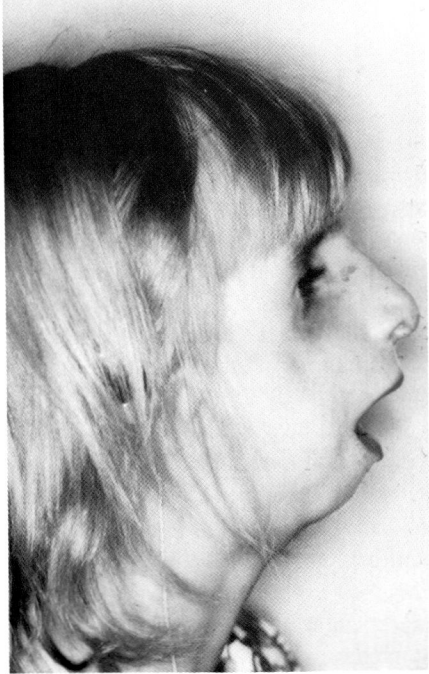

Fig. 1-16. Treacher Collins syndrome (mandibulofacial dysostosis). The patient had antimongoloid slanting of palpebral fissures, mild lower lid colobomas, partial absence of lower eyelashes, bilateral external ear dysplasia, conductive hearing loss, malar hypoplasia, mandibular hypoplasia, and cleft palate. (Courtesy of Dr. David Bixler, Department of Oral-Facial Genetics, Indiana University Medical Center, Indianapolis, Indiana.)

A syndrome similar to, and questionably distinct from, mandibulofacial dysostosis is the *otomandibular dysostosis of Konigsmark and Gorlin* (1976). This is an autosomal dominant disorder which includes prominent lop ears, long thin nares, micrognathia, and bilateral fixation of the stapes footplate. This is the only family described in the literature thus far.

The pathogenesis of both mandibulofacial dysostosis and Konigsmark-Gorlin otomandibular dysostosis may be explained by yet another animal model developed by Poswillo (1974). He found that the mechanism of malformation for syndromes such as these two was early destruction of the neural crest cells of the facial and auditory primordia which migrate to the 1st and 2nd branchial arches. This destruction, before migration is well underway, leads to the formation of a "vacuum" in the area of the otic cup into which the surrounding tissues flow. Consequently the developing otic pit moves upwards into the 1st arch region and relocates over the angle of the mandible. In addition, there is a symmetric overall hypoplasia of many of the derivatives of the 1st and 2nd branchial arch mesenchyme.

The next 2 groups of major external ear malformation syndromes, branchio-oto dysplasia and ear dysplasia-renal adysplasia, will be considered together because there is not yet complete agreement as to their boundaries.

Autosomal dominant branchio-oto-renal dysplasia (BOR) was originally delineated by Melnick et al (1975, 1976) as an additional entity in a group of syndromes that are characterized by ear malformations, cervical fistulas and conductive, mixed or sensorineural hearing loss. Their report concerned a 2-generation family of 9 individuals in which the father and 3 of the 6 living children all had: 1) a mixed hearing loss with a Mondini type cochlear malformation and stapes fixation; 2) cup-shaped, anteverted pinnae with bilateral prehelical pits; 3) bilateral branchial cleft fistulas; and 4) bilateral renal dysplasia and anomalies of the collecting system (Fig. 1-17). A 4th child, who died at 5 months of age, was reported to have branchial cleft fistulas and bilateral polycystic kidneys at autopsy. Subsequently, Fitch and Srolovitz (1976) and Fraser et al (1977) reported families with a similar pattern of anomalies. The family reported by Martins (1961) also appears to represent the BOR syndrome, although no mention is made of audiologic testing in any of the 3 affected persons.

Other families without known renal anomalies (branchial-oto-dysplasia) have previously been reported in which anomalies of the embryonic branchial arch system and deafness have been transmitted as an autosomal dominant with variable gene expression. Wildervanck (1962), McLaurin et al (1966), Rowley (1969), Karmody and Feingold (1974) and Bailleul et al (1972) reported families in which bilateral cervical fistulas, bilateral preauricular pits and malformed auricles were associated with a conductive or mixed hearing loss. The family of McLaurin et al (1966) also had one affected person with a bilateral sensorineural hearing loss. Bourguet et al (1966) described a family in which the mother and 6 offspring presented with branchial arch anomalies, facial paresis and deafness of all 3 types, conductive, mixed and sensorineural. Shenoi (1972) presented a kindred of 10 persons including 1 with bilateral preauricular pits, 1 with bilateral preauricular pits and tags with bilateral sensorineural deafness and 2 with bilateral preauricular pits and mixed deafness. Three of these had deformed auricles. Finally, Fourman and Fourman (1955) described a family in which 14 members in 3 generations had preauricular pits; of these, 3 had branchial fistulas and 12 had adult-onset deafness.

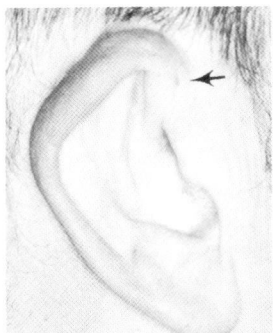

Fig. 1-17. Branchio-oto-renal dysplasia: the reported cases thus far have presented with A) malformed pinnas with or without preauricular pits, B) bilateral branchial cleft sinuses (infected in the picture shown here), and C) aplasias, hypoplasias, and dysplasias of the kidneys — the IVP pictured here shows a hypoplastic right kidney and ureter with the ureteropelvic junction peaked cranially, while the left kidney has a segmental hypoplasia with a sharply tapering configuration toward the superior pole, reduced parenchymal volume, and blunted calyceal fornices. (From Melnick M et al: Autosomal dominant branchiootorenal dysplasia. Birth Defects 11(5):121–128, 1975. With permission.)

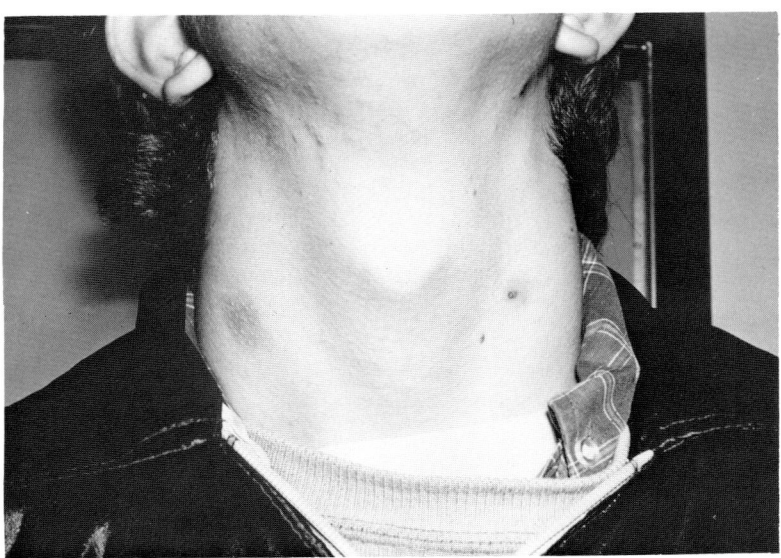

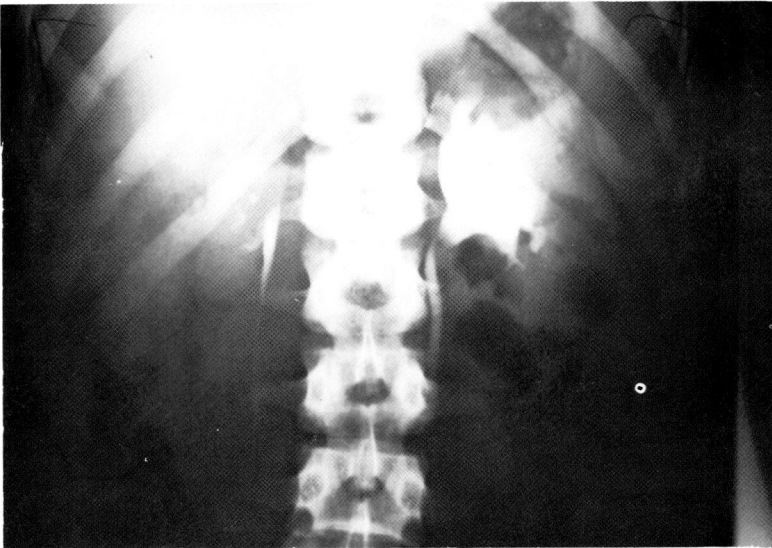

One other person had cervical fistulas only and deafness, and 2 others just had the deafness. All the deafness in this family was sensorineural.

The embryologic events common to the syndromes described above have been reviewed in a previous report (Melnick et al, 1976). At least one possible mechanism of malformation can be hypothesized from recent experimental evidence. Johnston (1975) has provided much evidence of dynamic ectomesenchymal migration from the neural crest over and around the head to provide connective tissue support to the face which until then is composed of essentially multiple bilamellar branchial membranes. The derivatives of this migrating neural crest are numerous. As pointed out above, the only major components of the face not of crest origin are the retina and lens, epithelial tissues, vascular endothelia and skeletal muscle. Ectomesenchymal deficiency in the area of the 1st and 2nd branchial arches will lead to external ear and ossicular anomalies, whereas deficiency of this tissue in the neck results in a branchial cleft fistula (Stark, 1973). There are 2 possible major consequences of ectomesenchymal deficiency: 1) the unreinforced bilamellar branchial membrane splits apart, or 2) there is disruption of highly coordinated inductive interactions. Either consequence may be associated with a constitutional deficiency of ectomesenchyme or late rather than normally programmed arrival of that tissue. This concept of ectomesenchymal integrity as a factor in malformations of the ear has been well documented in animal models by Poswillo (1973, 1974).

The renal dysplasia found in the BOR syndrome is most likely associated with an aberrant inductive interaction between the ureteric bud and the metanephrogenic mesenchymal mass (Gluecksohn-Waelsch, 1963). Again this may also arise because of a constitutional cell deficiency and/or late arrival of these cells. The association of such renal malformations with ear malformations has long been recognized (Hilson, 1957).

It is becoming increasingly apparent that cell interactions play a critical role in the choosing of new developmental pathways by embryonic cells and that genetically programmed cell surface components are instrumental in governing such cellular interrelationships. For example, the t^9 mutant in the mouse is associated with a failure of ectodermal cells to make the normal transition to mesoderm because of defective cell-cell recognition (Bennett, 1975). Thus, the embryologic events underlying the syndromes reported here, and perhaps the single genetic anomalies of the external ear and branchial clefts, may also represent a failure of directed cell movement and/or cellular spatial organization. Johnston (1975) seems to favor the idea that the branchial arch derivatives are more affected by defective crest migration. This could be associated with an alteration in the character of cell-cell recognition surface proteins as the result of a single gene mutation. The resultant abnormal cell numbers and/or arrangement in the mesenchymal components of the branchial arches, metanephrogenic masses, etc, could alter the temporal sequence of interactions between differentiated regions in their attempt to initiate secondary pattern formation.

There is now substantial evidence from the chick that the migration and spatial organization of large masses of cells depends upon the proteolytic cleavage of cell surface glycoproteins to form cell-associating molecules (Edelman, 1976). In the case of the BOR syndrome, the specific gene product would necessarily be an element common to the morphogenesis of the branchial, renal and auditory systems. Among other possibilities, this gene product might either be the cell surface glycoprotein or the proteolytic enzyme. In either case, it seems likely that much information could be obtained by employing an animal model system for demonstrating the extent of immunologic similarity, if any, between cell surface recognition antigens on those cells responsible for branchial, renal and auditory pattern formations.

A few studies of a similar nature have already been reported. Using immunochemical and immunohistochemical techniques in the rat and guinea pig, Quick et al (1973) were able to demonstrate evidence of a shared antigen between the kidney and the cochlea. This relationship appears to be particularly strong between the stria vascularis of the inner ear and the renal glomeruli (Arnold et al, 1976). Although these studies were done in adult animals, rather than in developing embryos, the results appear to constitute more than fortuitous support for the hypothesized mechanism of malformation in the BOR syndrome.

The two sons in the BOR family reported by Melnick et al (1978) and the daughter in the case reported by Fitch and Srolovitz (1976) raise an important diagnostic consideration in that they all present a pattern of anomalies characteristic of the "Potter syndrome." Buchta et al (1973) have designated this syndromic entity as a "symptomatic deformity complex" consisting of both malformations (micrognathia, pulmonary hypoplasia, ureto-bladder anomalies and occasionally cleft palate) and deformations (flat nose, large, flat auricles, talipes equinovarus and other limb anomalies), both of which are associated with oligohydramnios. This oligohydramnios may result from bilateral renal agenesis or severe dysplasia or from other causes of decreased amniotic fluid (Barr and Burdi, 1976). Buchta et al (1973) are careful to point out, and we would agree, that true auricular dysmorphogenesis, such as that described in the BOR family of Melnick et al (1978), Fitch and Srolovitz (1976), Warkany (1971, p. 1038) and case 3 of the Hilson (1957) report, are most often present in cases of renal agenesis associated with true multiple congenital anomaly syndromes. Such syndromes have been grouped into a genetically heterogeneous category called "hereditary renal adysplasia" (HRA), the adysplasia being a composite term for agenesis and dysplasia and implies predominantly asymmetric involvement or less commonly bilateral agenesis or symmetric degrees of dysplasia (Buchta et al, 1973).

Syndromes which would fall in the subcategory of HRA with ear malformations include the BOR syndrome (Melnick et al, 1975, 1976, 1978, Fitch and Srolovitz, 1976; Fraser et al, 1977; Martins, 1961; probably cases 1 and 2 Hilson, 1957), the dysplastic pinna-hypospadias-renal adysplasia syndrome (case 3, Hilson, 1957), the dysplastic pinna-polycystic kidney (Type II?) syndrome (case 4, Hilson, 1957), and probably the oto-renal-genital syndrome of Winter et al (1968). The first three syndromes are autosomal dominant with many overlapping features, and the extent to which they may represent the same entity or perhaps multiple allelism cannot be determined. The oto-renal-genital syndrome is most likely autosomal recessive.

Konigsmark and Gorlin (1976) have chosen to consider branchio-oto-renal dysplasia and branchio-oto dysplasia as a single disease entity. However, the clinical and experimental evidence to date would suggest otherwise. First, all the comparatively few well-documented cases of BOR syndrome (Melnick et al, 1975, 1976, 1978; Fitch and Srolovitz, 1976; Fraser et al, 1977) have had a significant sensorineural component to their hearing loss, whereas in branchio-oto-dysplasia this component may be lacking. Second, this sensorineural hearing loss in BOR syndrome has, with one exception (Fitch and Srolovitz, 1976), always been accompanied by macroscopic renal dysmorphology varying in severity from agenesis and cystic kidneys to so-called "silent" malformations. This has been so even in the family ascertained because of external ear anomalies rather than "silent" renal anomalies (Melnick et al, 1975, 1976; Fraser et al, 1977). Other families ascertained in this way and carefully studied have not been shown to have these renal anomalies (Melnick et al, 1978). Third, the experimental demonstration of a similar antigenicity of some components of the inner ear and kidney in other mammals makes the rather consistent observation of sensorineural deafness and renal anomalies in the BOR syndrome patients a reasonable phenotypic expectation given the mutation of a gene whose product is that shared antigen. Thus, although the anomalies of the auditory apparatus are often quite similar in the BOR and branchio-oto dysplasia syndromes, until demonstrated otherwise, one must assume we are dealing with 2 separate genetic diseases, one in which the gene product is critical for both renal and auditory development, and one in which it is critical for auditory development alone. When the fact that nearly 40% of the known offspring with BOR syndrome died within the first 6 months of life is considered, the importance of this distinction for genetic counseling should be obvious.

Finally, the within-family variability of expression of the branchial arch malformations (ie pinna anomalies, preauricular pits and tags, and cervical fistulas) has been quite remarkable. Nishimura and Okamoto (1976) maintain that at least the ear malformations appear to be variable expressions of the same dysmorphogenic event. This belief is strongly supported by the animal studies of Poswillo (1973). The same variable expressivity exists with regard to the type of deafness, particularly in branchio-oto dysplasia. Although the membranous labyrinth develops independently of both the external and middle ear, combined dysplasias of the 3 auditory components do occur with considerable frequency in these families. Even when this variable expressivity in most families is considered, there is probably still no justification for considering families with sensorineural deafness only (Fourman and Fourman, 1955) as yet a third entity, particularly in the absence of adequate examination of the kidneys.

It should be pointed out that, in addition to the primary branchio-oto dysplasia syndrome, there are at least 2 other syndromes that belong in this group, the autosomal recessive microtia-meatal atresia-conductive hearing loss syndrome (Ellwood et al, 1968) and the autosomal dominant Escher-Hirt syndrome characterized by hypertrophic ear lobes and conductive hearing loss due to malformation of the incudostapedial junction (Escher and Hirt, 1968).

The group labeled "variable system" syndromes is perhaps the most highly subjective. The sole criterion for inclusion was that the external ear malformations were so striking that their primacy in the syndrome was obvious. The group will be considered in alphabetic order:

1) *Auriculo-osteodysplasia* (Beals, 1967): a uniquely malformed ear characterized by a divided lobule, hip dysplasia, dysplasia of the capitellum with or without radial-head dislocation, short stature and autosomal dominant inheritance.

2) *Bixler syndrome* (Bixler et al, 1969): microtia, atresia of the external auditory canals, middle ear ossicle malformations, conductive deafness, mild frontonasal dysplasia (hypertelorism, bifid nasal tip, cleft lip and palate), short stature, renal ectopia, and hypoplasia of the thenar eminences of both hands. The inheritance is probably autosomal recessive. Johnston (1975) suggests that a blockage of crest-cell migration may be involved in the genesis of the frontonasal dysplasia. In this case the defect would be in the cells themselves, and such defective crest-cell migration probably accounts for the more caudal dysplasia (microtia and ossicle dysmorphia) as well.

3) *LADD syndrome* (Hollister et al, 1973): cup ears, conductive and sensorineural deafness, various digital anomalies, nasolacrimal atresia, enamel hypoplasia and other dental anomalies, and autosomal dominant inheritance.

4) *Mengel syndrome* (Mengel et al, 1969): variable external ear anomalies (hypoplasia, microtia, and lop), ossicle malformations, conductive hearing loss, mental retardation, heart murmur, hypogonadism, and cryptorchism. The inheritance pattern is autosomal recessive.

5) *Otocephaly anomaly* (Black et al, 1973): a failure of the developing auricles to move in a dorsolateral direction because of an associated agenesis or hypoplasia of the mandible. Consequently, the ears stay close to the midline of the neck and may fuse (synotia). Johnston (1975) believes the primary problem to be an interference with neural crest-cell migration to the distal end of the mandibular arch.

6) *Oto-facio-cervical syndrome* (Fara et al, 1967): cup ears, preauricular sinuses, branchial cleft sinuses, conductive hearing loss, weak neck musculature with sloping shoulders and depressed clavicles, hyporeflexia, and unilateral renal agenesis in one affected family member. The inheritance pattern is autosomal dominant.

7) *Townes-Brocks syndrome* (Townes and Brocks, 1972): lop ears, sensorineural deafness, imperforate anus, triphalangeal thumbs and other skeletal anomalies, and autosomal dominant inheritance.

In an attempt to provide an overview of the abnormal development of the external ear and branchial clefts, a brief synopsis of both individual malformations and the major syndrome groups has been presented. From the clinical and experimental evidence extant at this time, at least 2 conclusions may be drawn: 1) the within-family, and indeed "within-person," variabiliy of the external ear and/or branchial cleft anomalies is quite considerable, and it is apparent from the animal models and single gene syndromes that a single etiologic factor may be associated with a variety of ear malformations even in one individual; 2) the embryologic and teratologic evidence would seem to support the idea that external ear and branchial cleft malformations are associated with a breakdown in neural crest integrity, more often than not the result of aberrant crest-cell migration.

2. Epidemiology

THE NATURE OF PREVIOUS DATA

The focus of this chapter will be primarily on the descriptive epidemiologic studies of external ear and branchial cleft malformations that have been reported in the literature to date. Descriptive data can be found to a greater or lesser degree for the following parameters: incidence, race, ethnic and geographic distribution, sex distribution, laterality, and the association with other malformations. Although a number of studies are reported below, these vary in design and reliability. It should be remembered that there have been no specific major epidemiologic-genetic studies of branchial arch malformations to date. The data presented here derive from studies which for the most part focused on other major malformations. Some of the investigations were prospective while others were retrospective, depending on birth registries. Some studies had nearly complete ascertainment and others display varying degrees of incomplete ascertainment. The adherence to preestablished protocol varied and in at least one study (Marden et al, 1964) the interpretation of what constituted an anomaly changed during the course of the investigation. Finally, some studies were concerned with live births only, while others included fetal deaths. All this clearly demonstrates that it is difficult to make meaningful comparisons between studies. Nevertheless, these studies provide some useful baseline statistics from which etiologic hypotheses may be constructed and tested in more definitive studies.

INCIDENCE

The findings of a number of studies are listed in Table 2-1. The variation in incidence for the total of external ear malformations is quite striking, ranging from 2.41 to 88.40 per 10,000 births. This extreme heterogeneity is also found for the incidence of specific types of external ear malformations as well as

TABLE 2-1. Incidence Per 10,000 of External Ear and Branchial Cleft Malformations in Various Studies Worldwide

	Stevenson et al 1950 Boston MA	McIntosh et al 1954 New York NY	Marden et al 1964 Madison WI	Conway and Wagner 1965 New York NY	Stevenson et al 1966 Worldwide	Nelson and Forfar 1969 Edinburgh UK	Villumsen 1970 Copenhagen Denmark	CDC 1975 USA
Preauricular sinus	---	24.39	15.87	┤1.46├	---	5.75	0.00	---
Preauricular tag	---	29.62	27.20		*	20.74	44.66	5.58
Anotia/microtia	---	0.00	2.27	0.57	1.06	1.15	0.00	0.65
Other pinna malformations	---	5.23	43.06	0.78	*	2.30	3.27	---
Total ear malformations	2.41	59.24	88.40	2.81	8.90	29.94	47.93	---
Branchial cleft sinus	0.69	5.03	0.00	0.31	---	3.45	0.00	---

*Combined by Stevenson et al (1966 a and b) into one category and reflected in the total.

branchial cleft malformations. A good deal of this variation can certainly be attributed to variations in protocol design, diagnostic bias, diagnostic acumen, and other factors that alter the degree of reporting for a given malformation. On the other hand, it is also likely that at least part of the variation represents true differences in racial, ethnic and geographic frequencies.

Stevenson et al (1950) abstracted and analyzed the obstetric records of all mothers who gave birth to congenitally malformed infants, live or stillborn, in the Boston Lying-in Hospital during the years 1930 through 1941, together with the pediatric records of their live babies during the neonatal period. In all there were 677 malformed infants from 29,024 births during the study period. There were 658 malformed white infants, 18 black and 1 Chinese. Of the 677 infants there were 2 with branchial cleft sinuses and 7 with malformations of the external ear. The racial distribution or sex distribution of these infants was not listed. The retrospective design of this study precluded the establishment of uniform diagnostic criteria and reporting and this is apparently reflected in the extremely low incidence of external ear malformations as compared to other subsequent studies.

McIntosh et al (1954) conducted a prospective study of the outcome of 5,964 pregnancies at the Sloane Hospital for Women in New York City. The women were ascertained upon admission to the antepartum clinic over a period of 5 years beginning in October, 1946. These women were monitored through delivery and the infants were given a careful physical examination in the neonatal period by a pediatrician on the study team. Follow-up examinations were made at 6 and 12 months of age. Of the 5,739 deliveries in which the fetus weighed over 500 gm, 433 products of conception were found to have congenital malformations. Of these 433, there were 3 branchial cleft sinuses, 17 preauricular tags, 14 preauricular sinuses, and 3 other "minor" malformations of the external ear. No cases of microtia were listed. It is interesting to note that 1 case of preauricular tags was discovered by chance after the 1-year examination, pointing up the need for long-term follow-up in such studies. In fact less than 50% of the total number of malformations found among live-born infants were suspected or noted at birth. Although the racial distribution among the mothers was 55.8% white and 44.2% non-white, there was no analysis of each separate malformation by race. The same was true for sex of the infant.

Marden et al (1964) over a 2-year period from June, 1960 to May, 1962 examined 4,412 newborn infants at St. Mary's Hospital in Madison, Wisconsin. The infants were examined on the 1st or 2nd postnatal day. For this reason many stillborn babies were not examined. No babies were examined for 2 two-month periods and 1 one-month period. Decisions as to what constituted an anomaly were subject to continued review and some variants were scored after the study was under way and thus for only some of the total population (Hook et al, 1976). Except for 9 black and 15 oriental infants the entire population was white. A more extensive presentation of the "minor" anomalies in this study population can be found in Hook et al (1976). Among those with malformations, 12 had preauricular tags, 7 preauricular sinuses, 19 with other external ear malformations, and 1 with microtia in the absence of multiple major malformations. There were no branchial cleft fistulas recorded.

Conway and Wagner (1965), in order to determine the birth incidence of selected head and neck malformations, recorded the congenital anomalies reported on birth certificates of the city of New York from 1952 through 1962. In all, there were 1,823,244 births during the 11-year study period and 21,804 malformed children, an incidence of 1.2%. Included in the total malformed were 267 infants with preauricular sinuses and/or tags, 104 with anotia/microtia, 142 with other external ear malformations, and 56 with branchial cleft malformations. These incidence figures are considerably lower than those found in the prospective New York study of McIntosh et al (1954). This can probably be accounted for by the retrospective design and the fact that all recorded observations were restricted to the neonatal period. Race, ethnic and sex distributions are provided in this study and will be discussed below.

Stevenson et al (1966 a and b) reported a WHO study of consecutive births in 24 centers in 16 countries. Data were collected prospectively on the outcomes of 421,781 pregnancies (416,695 singletons and 5,086 multiple births). The data were tabulated with respect to the occurrence and type of congenital malformations found in stillborn and live-born infants. The data for each birth were limited to that which could fit on a 5 X 8 inch check list with little room for elaborate explanation. Starting on a fixed date in each hospital every live birth and stillbirth of over 28 weeks gestation was recorded during a period of 3 years from October, 1961 to December, 1964. Although there was a uniform recording system and a fairly standardized classification of malformations, the diagnostic criteria and interests varied from center to center and this was particularly evident for the minor malformations. Anotia/microtia was classified as a miscellaneous major malformation and there were 44 such nonsyndromic cases recorded. Those ear malformations which were classified as minor included preauricular tags and other types of pinna anomalies. In all there were 327 such anomalies recorded. Curiously there were no preauricular sinuses noted in any of the 24 centers. In spite of its many shortcomings, the study does allow for some meaningful comparisons by race, ethnic group, and sex.

The study by Nelson and Forfar (1969) covered a 2-year period in which all babies born in 3 maternity units in Edinburgh, Scotland were examined for congenital malformations. The observation period during which malformations could have been detected was the first 10 days of postnatal life. Nearly all examinations were completed by a single examiner in order to maintain uniformity. Of the 8,684 deliveries 470 infants had congenital malformations, major and minor. Of these, 1 had microtia, 5 preauricular sinuses, 18 preauricular tags, and 2 other minor external ear malformations. Three infants had branchial cleft fistulas. No mention is made of race and it is assumed that all infants were white. Sex distribution was also not mentioned.

The data of Villumsen (1970) were collected from 1959 to 1962 as part of the prospective Copenhagen Perinatal Project in which 9,180 children were born (8,833 singletons and 173 multiple births). The recorded malformations include only those which were observed within the first 5 days of postnatal life or at autopsy in the case of stillborn and neonatal death. In all there were 350 children with a total of 582 malformations, 229 children having a single malformation only. Of these 350 children, 41 had nonsyndromic preauricular tags and 3 others had other nonsyndromic external ear anomalies. There were no preauricular or branchial cleft sinuses recorded. The population was white and the sex is recorded for each infant.

The Birth Defect Monitoring Program (Center for Disease Control, 1975) is a collaborative effort involving 2 governmental agencies and 2 private, nonprofit organizations. Its primary purpose is to monitor the incidence of birth defects and other newborn conditions. Discharge abstracts are coded by a hospital's medical records department staff and submitted regularly for data processing. Included are abstracts for all live and stillborn infants delivered in each of 1,200 participating hospitals. While these data are not a random sample of United States births, it nevertheless represents the largest single source of uniformly collected and coded discharge data on birth defects among newborn infants. Maternal data, however, are not routinely available through this system. Obviously in a data source this large uniformity of diagnosis and interest is out of the question and this raises a serious problem for malformations in which the diagnostic criteria are in some dispute and even more particularly for "minor" malformations. Between April, 1974 and March, 1975 there were 975,005 births reported and of these 544 were recorded as having preauricular tags. This incidence is less than 1/5 that reported by McIntosh et al (1954) in New York and Marden et al (1964) in Wisconsin and suggests serious underreporting of this "minor" anomaly.

With regard to birth incidence of external ear and branchial cleft malformations, it can be stated with certainty that the data are confusing. On the basis of prospective design, uniformity of protocol, completeness of ascertainment and follow-up examinations over the first year of life, it would be reasonable to expect that the most accurate incidence figures available prior to the present study are those of McIntosh et al (1954). The 95% confidence limits for the New York incidence of preauricular sinuses lies between 11.6 and 37.2 per 10,000, for preauricular tags between 15.5 and 43.7 per 10,000, and for other minor external ear anomalies and branchial cleft sinuses between virtually 0.0 and 11.2

36 / INTRODUCTION

per 10,000. Because of their study design and the demographic make-up of their population, there is a good chance that the actual U.S. incidence may also lie between these limits.

RACE, ETHNIC AND GEOGRAPHIC DISTRIBUTION

Racial and ethnic differences in incidences of many human disorders are known to exist and have received considerable attention in recent years (McKusick, 1974; Adam, 1974). Quelprud (1940) examined the village population of Hessen, Germany and found the frequency of preauricular sinuses to be 1.7%. Ewing (1946) in a "cursory" examination of 3,500 British naval recruits found 31 or 0.9% with preauricular sinuses while Gualandri (1969) found 321 preauricular sinuses in a study of 29,309 Milan, Italy school children, or a frequency of 1.1%. Stannus (1914), in an examination of 6,491 Bantus in what was then Nyasaland, found 292 or 4.5% with preauricular sinuses. The frequency in oriental populations has been reported by Congdon et al (1932) to be 4-6% and by Ride in 1935 to be 10-14%. In a study of Hamilton County, Ohio school children, 0.9% of the white and 5.2% of the black children were found to have preauricular sinuses (Selkirk, 1935). For preauricular tags the frequency has ranged from 1.5% in the American population (Altmann, 1951) to 0.2% in a population of 7,537 school children in Marburg, Germany (Ostmann, 1903). Aase and Tegtmeier (1977) presented data showing an 8-fold increase in the frequency of microtia among American Indians as compared with other racial groups in the United States. This supported a similar finding by Jaffe (1969). Selkirk (1935) found the frequency of branchial cleft malformations to be 0.5% among white Hamilton County, Ohio school children but 0.0% among black children. Although these various data sources show some distinct racial and regional differences, they unfortunately represent the results of either retrospective ascertainment from registries or prevalence measures. The measure of choice for congenital malformations is clearly the incidence rate for it provides a direct measure of the risk, or the probability of occurrence of a specific malformation (Myrianthopoulos, 1977). Other epidemiologic measures cannot do this except by indirect estimate.

Although relatively few data exist for the birth incidence of external ear malformations in various racial and ethnic groups, it may be somewhat instructive to look at those studies outlined in Table 2-1. The most reliable studies, based on protocol design, for preauricular sinuses and tags are those of McIntosh et al (1954), Nelson and Forfar (1969), and Villumsen (1970). In the racially mixed New York City population (McIntosh et al, 1954) the incidence of preauricular tags was 1½ times greater than in the white population in Edinburgh, Scotland (Nelson and Forfar, 1969) but 1½ times lower than in the white population in Copenhagen, Denmark (Villumsen, 1970). As we proceed eastward from New York City to Edinburgh to Copenhagen, the incidence of preauricular sinuses falls off dramatically, being 4 times greater in New York than in Edinburgh (Copenhagen being 0%). This may be a reflection of the large proportion of blacks in the New York study but unfortunately McIntosh et al (1954) do not provide a tabulation by race of their data. Support for this explanation comes from a study by Simpkiss and Lowe (1961) in which they examined 2,068 consecutive newborn babies between December, 1956 and September, 1957 in Mulago Hospital, Kampala, Uganda. The incidence of preauricular sinuses in this black African newborn population was 222.43 per 10,000 (or 2.2%) nearly 10 times greater than the New York study and 39 times greater than the Edinburgh study. It is interesting to note that incidences of preauricular tags (24.17 per 10,000) and other pinna malformations (9.67 per 10,000) are similar to those found in the other prospective studies. For completeness, it should also be noted here that the retrospective study by Conway and Wagner (1965) found the incidence of preauricular sinuses and tags and other external ear malformations to be uniformly higher in whites than in blacks, although not by much.

The most accurate assessment we have thus far regarding the ethnicity of anotia/microtia is the worldwide study reported by Stevenson et al (1966 a and b). The incidences by race and country are listed in Table 2-2. Mestizos in Latin America are of mixed racial background, Spanish or Portuguese and American Indian. The incidence of anotia/microtia in the 4 Mestizos populations of 10,000 persons or greater (Bogota, Medellin, Mexico City, and Panama City) are comparable with that found in similar size populations of orientals (Kuala Lumpur, Singapore, and Manila) and both are lower than many of the large white populations (Melbourne, Santiago, Czechoslovakia and Johannesburg). There appears to be no particular geographic clustering of high incidence, the areas of unusually high incidence being Australia, Malaysia, South Africa, Czechoslovakia and Chile. Interestingly enough these high incidences are due to affected white persons. Based on these data, the 8-fold increase in American Indians found by Aase and Tegtmeier (1977) certainly requires confirmation with prospective incidence data.

SEX DISTRIBUTION

Differential sex distributions are well known for many of the common malformations in man, eg facial clefting, pyloric stenosis, neural tube malformations, etc. Without providing either references or data, Smith (1976) claims that preauricular sinuses are twice as common in females as in males. The study by Quelprud (1940) in Hessen, Germany would support this contention, the 13 cases being distributed as 4 males and 9 females. However, in the Madison study (Marden et al, 1964; Hook et al, 1976), the male/female ratio for this malformation was 1.3. Similarly, in the school survey in Ohio (Selkirk, 1935) the

TABLE 2-2. Incidences Per 10,000 of Microtia in the WHO Study by Ethnic Group and Race*

	White	Black	Oriental	Mestizos	Total
Melbourne, Australia (I)	1.27	---	---	---	1.27]**
Melbourne, Australia (II)	10.49	---	---	---	10.49
Sao Paulo, Brazil	1.24	1.60	0.00	---	1.37
Santiago, Chile	3.41	---	0.00	---	3.34
Bogota, Colombia	0.00	0.00	0.00	1.08	1.05
Medellin, Colombia	0.00	0.00	0.00	0.59	0.48
Various cities, Czechoslovakia	1.97	---	---	---	1.97
Alexandria, Egypt	0.00	---	---	---	0.00
Hong Kong	0.00	---	0.00	---	0.00
Bombay, India	0.50	---	---	---	0.50
Calcutta, India	0.52	---	0.00	---	0.52
Kuala Lumpur, Malaysia	4.57	---	1.74	---	2.52
Singapore, Malaysia	0.00	---	1.09	---	1.01
Mexico City, Mexico (I)	0.00	---	0.00	1.21	1.20
Mexico City, Mexico (II)		not given by race			0.71
Belfast, N. Ireland		not given by race			0.00
Panama City, Panama	0.00	0.00	0.00	1.67	1.25
Manila, Philippines	---	---	1.02	---	1.02
Cape Town, S. Africa	---	0.00	---	---	0.00
Johannesburg, S. Africa	1.77	---	---	---	1.77
Pretoria, S. Africa	---	0.00	---	---	0.00
Madrid, Spain	0.00	---	---	---	0.00
Ljubljana, Yugoslavia	1.11	---	---	---	1.11
Zagreb, Yugoslavia	0.00	---	---	---	0.00

*As computed by this author from the data of Stevenson et al (1966 a and b).
**Combined Australia = 4.28 per 10,000.

male/female ratio of affected persons was virtually the same as the ratio in the whole study population.

In the Madison study (Hook et al, 1976), the male/female ratio for preauricular tags was 1.4 and in a larger sample (Villumsen, 1970) the ratio for preauricular sinuses and tags combined was 1.3.

In the prospective data series presented by Stevenson et al (1966 a and b) the male/female ratio for anotia/microtia was 1.2 and in the retrospective study by Conway and Wagner (1965) the ratio was 1.1. On the other hand, Aase and Tegtmeier (1977) maintain that there is a "marked predilection for the male sex."

The male/female ratios for all external ear malformations combined was 1.11 in the study by Marden et al (1964), 1.22 in the WHO study by Stevenson et al (1966 a and b), 1.32 in the Danish study by Villumsen (1970), and 1.26 in the New

York study by Conway and Wagner (1965). The male/female ratio for branchial cleft malformations was 1.55 in the study by Conway and Wagner (1965).

LATERALITY

Very few data are available with regard to laterality, that is data from population-based prospective studies. In the data presented on anotia/microtia by Stevenson et al (1966a and b) 13 of the 44 cases (30%) were bilateral. Of the 31 unilateral cases, the laterality (right or left) was recorded for 27. The right/left ratio $16/11 = 1.5$ was not significantly different from 1 ($\chi_1^2 = 0.93$). This differs considerably from the data of Aase and Tegtmeier (1977) which shows a "marked predilection for the right side."

Altmann (1951) states that preauricular tags are more frequently unilateral than bilateral. This is supported by recent data. In the Villumsen (1970) series of 41 cases, 3 were bilateral and 38 were unilateral being equally divided between the right and left side. In the prevalence study in Marburg, Germany by Ostmann (1903) all 12 cases of preauricular tags were unilateral, 5 right and 7 left.

For estimates of laterality with regard to preauricular sinuses we must look to the prevalence studies. In the Ohio series reported by Selkirk (1935) 77% of the cases were unilateral, the right/left ratio being 1.2. In the Hessen, Germany series of 13 cases, 6 were bilateral, 3 were unilateral right, and 4 were unilateral left. In the African series reported by Stannus (1914) 83% of the cases were unilateral, the right/left ratio again being 1.2.

In summary, these data indicate that for all external ear malformations the tendency is for unilaterality. A strong predilection for one or the other side seems generally to be absent from these data.

ASSOCIATED MALFORMATIONS

There exist many instances in which a given single malformation may be associated with one or more other malformations. A rather prominent "coupling" of this type is orofacial clefting and clubfoot. Some data of a similar nature also exist for external ear malformations.

Of the 44 cases reported by Villumsen (1970), 3 (6.82%) had one other malformation and these were all of the toes. This was nearly 10 times greater than the overall frequency (0.69%) of toe malformations found in this population. Similarly, in the study by Nelson and Forfar (1969) 2 of the 25 ear malformations cases (or 8%) had a "limb" anomaly as compared to 1.2% in the overall study population. In addition, 5 other infants with ear malformations had skin nevi of various types, an incidence of 20% as compared to about a 0.7% overall incidence for such nevi.

In light of the experimental animal data presented by Poswillo (1973), the finding of a high incidence of limb malformations is not surprising. Apparently drugs which induce hematoma formation in the region of the branchial arches also induce localized, destructive hematomas in the limb (DE Poswillo, personal communication). The increased incidence of skin nevi is not quite as easy to explain but perhaps it is related to the common origin of the ectomesenchyme of the auricular hillocks and the melanocytes, namely the neural crest.

SYNDROME INCIDENCE

Except for the more obvious entities, specific syndromes are not usually presented as such in incidence studies of congenital malformations. Three of the syndromes for which some data exist are the first and second branchial arch syndrome, the synotia anomaly, and the Townes-Brocks syndrome.

By reviewing the records of 23,898 births at the University of Michigan Medical Center from 1943 through 1962 and 15,594 births at St. Joseph Mercy Hospital in Ann Arbor from 1957 through 1963, Grabb (1965) calculated the birth incidence of the first and second branchial arch syndrome to be 1 in 5,642 births. Using the rather cursory descriptions for multiple malformation cases reported in the WHO study (Stevenson et al, 1966a and b), one finds 3 cases of probable Townes-Brocks syndrome and 3 cases of the synotia anomaly, a birth incidence for each of these syndromes of about 1 in 139,000 births.

SUMMARY

The prospective birth incidences of various external ear and branchial cleft malformations, as estimated by a number of studies, are considerably heterogeneous (Table 2-1). There appear to be real racial and ethnic differences for these malformations. The sex distribution of these malformations is about 1.25. Most cases are unilateral, the right/left ratio being about 1.35. Two studies suggest that limb and pigmentation anomalies are more frequently associated with an isolated external ear malformation than would be expected on the basis of the general population incidences.

3. Etiology

EXTERNAL EAR AND BRANCHIAL CLEFT MALFORMATIONS AND SINGLE GENE MUTATIONS

When McKusick published his first catalog of Mendelian Inheritance in Man in 1966, he listed 1,487 phenotypic entities, 837 autosomal dominant, 531 autosomal recessive, and 119 X-linked. In the latest (5th) edition (McKusick, 1978), he lists 2,811 phenotypic entities, 1,489 autosomal dominant, 1,117 autosomal recessive, and 205 X-linked. This represents approximately a 90% increase in just 12 years. Although seemingly large, the total number of loci presently identified through phenotypic aberration represents a very small proportion of the total number of loci present in man's functional genome. No attempt will be made here to detail every known mutant that is associated with an external ear or branchial cleft malformation. Instead, we have chosen to outline what we consider to be the major single external ear and branchial cleft malformations and syndromes which involve such malformations that are associated with single gene mutations. We make no claim to having constructed the definitive list.

McKusick (1978) lists ear pits as an autosomal dominant trait (Catalog #12870). To be sure there have been numerous reports of multigeneration pedigrees with this malformation (Kindred, 1921; Whitney, 1939; Quelprud, 1940; Connon, 1941; McDonough, 1941; Stiles, 1945; Gualandri, 1969). These pedigrees display vertical and male-to-male transmission through 3 and 4 generations. There is, however, a number of consistent but atypical features in most reported families. First, there are numerous instances of one and sometimes two (Whitney, 1939) skipped generations. This incomplete penetrance is perhaps most graphically illustrated in the family reported by McDonough (1941). Monozygotic twins (by physiognomy) were born to an unaffected mother, 1 of the twins having an ear pit on the left. The *affected twin* subsequently married an unaffected woman and had *2 unaffected sons*. The *unaffected twin* married an unaffected woman and had *1 affected son* (bilateral ear pits). An unaffected maternal aunt of these twins had an affected son (unilateral left ear pit) and 3 other unaffected children. The maternal uncle of these twins was also affected (bilateral ear pits). Stiles (1945) in an analysis of 5 large, multigeneration families has estimated the penetrance to be about 50%. On the other hand, Gualandri (1969) using 93 families, including 2° relatives, estimates the penetrance to be 85% and the gene frequency 0.5%.

Second, there is considerable variation within sibships and between generations with regard to laterality. A good example is the family presented by Whitney (1939). A male with a unilateral left ear pit had a son with bilateral ear pits and 2 other unaffected children. The bilaterally affected son had 3 affected children out of 4, 2 with bilateral ear pits and 1 with a unilateral left ear pit. In the Connon (1941) pedigree, two sibs had unilateral ear pits but on different sides. Another good example is the McDonough (1941) pedigree described above. In the large pedigrees reported by Stiles (1945) there was unilateral expression in 22 of the 38 persons showing the trait.

Third, it is interesting to note that the frequency of a positive family history in a series of independently ascertained cases is quite low. In the Ohio series collected by Selkirk (1935) only 10% had a positive family history and in the sample of British naval recruits collected by Ewing (1946) only 3% had a positive family history. This finding may reflect poor proband recall, the decreased penetrance, and/or a high incidence of phenocopies, new mutations, etc.

Another interesting type of ear pit which is inherited as an autosomal dominant trait is the ear lobe pit or "congenitally pierced ears." Edmonds and Keeler (1940) reported 2 large families, the second one displaying skipped generations. In its typical form this malformation is expressed as a round or lenticular pit about a millimeter deep, situated in the middle of the lateral surface of the lobe of the ear, associated with a similar pit at a corresponding position on the medial surface of the lobe. Interestingly enough Stiles (1945) wrote: "The similarity between congenital sinuses of the lobe and the sinuses which result from perforations for rings is so great that the question of the inheritance of an acquired character has been raised."

At the turn of the century Ostmann (1903) published 2 pedigrees of persons with preauricular tags. There were skipped generations in both kindreds. Similarly other pedigrees showing dominance and sometimes incomplete penetrance were published by Siemens (1921), Jenkins (1928), and Brander (1939). Brander (1939), after reviewing the literature to that time, concluded that the trait had a "dominant predisposition with variegated penetration." As with preauricular pits, the pedigree presented by Brander (1939) shows a mother with a unilateral right ear tag having 2 out of 4 affected children, both with bilateral ear tags.

McKusick (1978) lists the "cup ear" malformation as an autosomal dominant trait (Catalog #12860). Potter (1937) reported 5 generations of a family in which 22 individuals had bilateral cup ears. Since that report, Peterson and Schimke (1968), Rogers (1968) and others have reported similar families. The penetrance seems to be nearly complete in the families thus far reported and the phenotypic expression is rather uniform.

Branchial cleft malformations have also been listed by McKusick (1978) as a confirmed autosomal dominant trait. Three generation kindreds with complete penetrance have been reported by Wheeler et al (1958) and Muckle (1961).

From the discussion thus far one could get the impression that each of these traits is etiologically distinct, but this is likely not to be the case. There are numerous reports in which two or more of these traits appear within the same nuclear family and sometimes in the same person. Ruttin (1927) reported a family in which a woman with a left preauricular pit had 2 children with right-sided preauricular pits and 1 child with a right-sided preauricular tag. In the family reported by Muckle (1961) a woman with bilateral 2nd branchial cleft fistulas had 1 son with a left preauricular sinus and bilateral 2nd branchial cleft fistulas, and another son with a left preauricular sinus and bilateral 1st and 2nd branchial cleft fistulas. The other 5 affected persons in this kindred had 2nd branchial cleft fistulas without preauricular sinuses. A similar family has been reported by Hunter (1974). In the kindred with "congenitally pierced ears" reported by Edmonds and Keeler (1940), the proband sibship had one sib with ear lobe sinuses, and another with ear lobe sinuses and moderate microtia, a phenotype identical to the paternal great-uncle. In this same family a sibship of 1st cousins to the proband had 2 children with ear lobe sinuses and 1 with preauricular sinuses without ear lobe sinuses. Finally, Rogers (1968) describes 2 brothers, 1 with bilateral protruding ears, and the other with microtia of the right ear and a protruding left ear. In a second family the proband has bilateral cup ears, and his sister and father have bilateral protruding ears. Obviously the extent of this intrafamilial phenotypic variation is considerable and quite similar to that seen in many of the syndromes described in Chapter 1. This phenomenon raises serious doubt as to whether there really are distinct genetic mutations for each separate phenotypic character. Perhaps we are witnessing, instead, intrafamilial genetic and/or environmental modification of only one or two distinct mutations for nonsyndromic external ear dysmorphogenesis.

Let us turn now to monogenic syndromes. The listing that follows is designed to be a further guide to appreciating the scope of single gene etiologies vis-a-vis external ear malformations. Each syndrome designation is followed by the currently understood pattern of inheritance and the most frequent external ear malformation. For the complete phenotypic description of these syndromes, the reader is referred to Bergsma (1973), Gorlin et al (1976), Smith (1976), Warkany (1971) and the other cited references. Additional syndromes may be found in Chapter 1 of this presentation. It should be emphasized that, as with all features in most syndromes, external ear malformations are not invariably found in the syndromes enumerated below. However, they are frequently found.

AD = Autosomal Dominant; AR = Autosomal Recessive; XL = X-linked
    Aarskog syndrome – XL: lop, protruding
    Acrocephalopolydactylous dysplasia – AR: dysplastic (Elejalde et al, 1977)
    Ampola syndrome; ?AD or XL: cupped (Ampola, 1974)
    Armendares syndrome; ?AR or XL: cupped (Armendares et al, 1975)
    Auriculo-polysyndactyly syndrome – AD: lobule cleft or nodule (Goldberg and Pashayan, 1976)
    Blepharophimosis syndrome – AD: cupped
    Carpenter syndrome – AR; preauricular fistulas
    Contractural arachnodactyly syndrome – AD: "crumpled" helix

44 / INTRODUCTION

    Cryptophthalmos syndrome—AR: cupped, cryptotia
    Diastrophic dwarfism—AR: hypertrophic ear cartilage
    Dubowitz syndrome—AR: protruding
    Focal dermal hypoplasia syndrome—XL: dysplastic
    Galloway-Mowat syndrome—AR: macrotia (Shapiro et al, 1976)
    Harrod-Keele-Howard syndrome—?AR or XL: macrotia, cupped (Harrod et al, 1977)
    KBG syndrome—AR: helix and anthelix dysplasia (Herrmann et al, 1975)
    Lenz microphthalmia syndrome—XL: dysplastic, hypoplastic, protruding
    Maxillofacial dysostosis—AD: cup, dysplastic (Melnick and Eastman, 1977)
    Meckel-Gruber syndrome—AR: variable dysplasias
    Multiple lentigines syndrome—AD: protruding
    Odontotrichomelic hypohidrotic dysplasia—AR: macrotia, protruding
    Orofaciodigital II syndrome—AR: cup, protruding
    Otodental dysplasia—AD: lop, protruding
    Pena-Shokeir syndrome—AR: dysplastic (Pena and Shokeir, 1976)
    Roberts syndrome—AR: dysplastic lobule
    Saethre-Chotzen syndrome—AD: prominent crus
    Say syndrome—AD: macrotia
    Seckel syndrome—AR: hypoplastic or absent lobule
    Trichorhinophalangeal syndrome—AD: macrotia, protruding

EXTERNAL EAR MALFORMATIONS AND CHROMOSOMAL ABERRATIONS

With the advent of new staining techniques in the early part of this decade, the number of detectable chromosomal aberrations has grown to almost intellectually unmanageable proportions. It is certain that with even more refined techniques this number will grow immeasurably. Many of these chromosomal anomalies are associated with rather unique and classic phenotypes but even so there are great overlaps of phenotypic expression between them all.

It is not the purpose of this chapter to discuss each known chromosomal anomaly that is associated with an external ear malformation. Nevertheless, it would be helpful here to look at a number of the more well-known chromosomal aberrations and the external ear malformations associated with them. The listing that follows has been compiled from Bergsma (1973), Borgaonkar et al (1976), Gorlin et al (1976), Smith (1976), and Warkany (1971). The nomenclature follows the recommendations of the Paris Conference (1972). It should be noted that the trisomy designations +13, +18 and +21 include the partial trisomies that result from unbalanced translocations.

  A) Preauricular sinus: 4p−; +21; +22
  B) Preauricular tags: 4p−; 5p−; +13; +18; +22

C) Macrotia, mild-to-moderate microtia, cup, lop, protruding and other auricular hillock dysplasias: 1q+; 4p-; 4p+; 5p-; r(6); 7q+; +8; 9p-; 9p+; 10p+; 10q+; 11p+; 11q+; +13; 13q-; r(13); 14q+; +18; 18p-; 18q-; r(18); +20; +21; 21q-; +22; 22q-; triploidy; XO; XXXY

It is obvious from this listing that the etiologic heterogeneity, vis-a-vis chromosomal aberrations, for a given type of pinna dysmorphogenesis is considerable. Conversely, the phenotypic variability, vis-a-vis external ear malformations, associated with any single chromosomal aberration is also considerable. For example, deletion of the short arm of chromosome 4 and complete or partial trisomy of chromosome 22 can be expressed phenotypically as preauricular sinuses, preauricular tags, pinna dysplasias, or as any combination of these 3 anomalies. This raises the question again whether it is tenable to view these genetic abnormalities as being associated with a unique auricular phenotype (eg ear tags) as opposed to an association with external ear dysmorphogenesis in general.

Utilizing phenotype-karyotype correlations in groups of patients with particular chromosomal deletions (deletion mapping), may someday lead to the assigning of loci for external ear development to particular chromosomes. Especially relevant here is the assignment by Noel et al (1976) of observed external ear malformations to a specific region (q22) of chromosome 13. It should be remembered that assignment of a phenotypic trait such as pinna development to the q22 region of chromosome 13 does not negate the probability that other loci on other chromosomes are also associated with pinna development. This is particularly obvious since such malformations are known to be associated with many other chromosome abnormalities. For example, macrotia is found in those patients with trisomy for the q21 to q31 region of chromosome 7, and pinna dysplasia is found in those patients with trisomy for the p11 to pter or q24 to q26 regions of chromosome 10 (Borgaonkar et al, 1976).

Finally, it should be noted that there is a striking similarity between the appearance of those children with autosomal dominant branchio-oto-renal dysplasia who have died in the neonatal period (Fitch and Srolovitz, 1976; Melnick et al, 1978) and a child reported with full trisomy 11 (Blair, 1976).

ENVIRONMENTAL ETIOLOGIES: AN INTRODUCTION

An environmental agent which is present during the critical periods of development and can be demonstrated to have a statistically significant, nonrandom association with a particular congenital malformation or set of malformations is termed an *environmental teratogenic agent* or *teratogen* (Shepard, 1973). These may include chemicals, pharmaceuticals, xrays, infectious agents, maternal pathophysiologic disorders, etc. Although Shepard (1973) lists over 600 such agents in his Catalog of Teratogenic Agents, only a handful are known to be unquestionably associated with human congenital malformations. This is not to minimize their importance as etiologic agents. The problem, however, lies in gathering incontrovertible evidence that a particular environmental agent is, in fact, teratogenic. Since the imperative avoidance of particular environmental agents during gestation may have serious economic consequences for a community or an individual (vis factory closures or restricted job opportunities) or present difficult moral and ethical questions regarding abortion for women who require long-term medication for a chronic disease, it is incumbent upon investigators to provide at least reasonably certain evidence for a claim of teratogenicity. The nature of human reproductive habits, sociocultural practices and gestation time often make the gathering of relevant prospective data more than formidable.

Before moving on to a consideration of specific environmental influences on human external ear development, a few words of explanation would be helpful. The next several sections on environmental etiologies deal primarily with either well-established or reasonably certain teratogens that may be associated with human external ear dysmorphology. The decision was made to refrain from examining suspected but poorly documented teratogens in an attempt to avoid the confusion and almost certain misinterpretations that result from such discussions. Most of the teratogens in this "suspected" class have been so labeled on the basis of a few individual case reports which purport an association between a particular environmental agent and a particular malformation. The inherent bias in such reporting should be obvious and the clinician should not accept this in any way as sufficient documentation. The only cautious exception to this is the case in which the agent and the malformation are so rare that the co-occurrence of these two in several reported cases is beyond all reasonable probability of coincidence. Such cases will undoubtedly be quite rare in themselves.

THE PLACENTA AND FETAL MEMBRANES

It should come as no surprise that the placenta and fetal membranes are of primary importance in controlling the fetal environment. While there are no placental abnormalities that have been positively associated with external ear malformations, it is likely that a number of pathologic conditions which affect the placenta result in fetal restraint and subsequent growth retardation (Poswillo, 1976). These include velamentous insertion of the cord, single umbilical artery, circumvallation, placental infections, tumors and infarcts (Benirschke 1975). To date, the precise consequences of those anomalies which contribute to placental dysfunction are not known but it is not unreasonable to speculate, for example, that hypoxia might be one of them. Regarding the hemorrhage hypothesis for the 1st and 2nd branchial arch syndrome (Poswillo, 1973), Poswillo (1975) favors the idea that it derives from the effect of a hypoxic hypertensive episode on the inherent weakness in the junction of the hyoid and ventropharyngeal arteries when they anastomose.

One of the most bizarre and graphic etiologies of external ear malformation is the formation of the amniotic or Streeter bands. These aberrant amniotic tissue bands range from filamentous strands or 2-3 mm wide bands of tissue to fusiform peduncles up to 20 mm in length (Jones, 1975). The speculations regarding the pathogenesis of these bands have ranged from an early defect of the ectoderm affecting both the amnion and the embryonic disk (Streeter, 1930) to early amniotic rupture or separation from the chorion followed by fetal swallowing of the fibrous band (Torpin, 1968). Regardless of the pathogenesis, these bands are often associated with a recognizable pattern of malformations including encephalocele, microcephaly, and other skull and scalp defects, bizarre facial and auricular clefts, nasal and ocular defects, and limb anomalies that include amputation, constriction or pseudosyndactyly (Broome et al, 1976). The incidence of this amniotic band syndrome has been estimated to be 1-3 cases per 28,000 births (Hanson and Freeman, 1975). This syndrome has been sporadic in occurrence and the recurrence risk in subsequent sibs would be considerably less than 1%. It is for this reason that this syndrome must be carefully differentiated from isolated anencephaly, isolated clefts of the lip and/or palate and such syndromes as the Meckel-Gruber syndrome.

Jones (1975) contends that the findings in these children are secondary to the destructive and disruptive forces of the aberrant tissue bands, beginning at least prior to 32 days of fetal age. Citing the recent work of Malcolm Johnston (1975) which demonstrates that neural crest cells migrate from the neural folds to form the early mesenchyme of the developing branchial arches, Jones (1975) states that early interference with this neural crest migration is probably the mechanism of malformation for many of the craniofacial anomalies in the amniotic band syndrome.

INFECTIOUS AGENTS

Although infectious agents have not been specifically associated with pinna malformations, it should be noted that as yet unknown endogenous maternal viruses may also influence development. The recent work of Mayer et al (1974) gives support to this possibility. The endogenous virus particles, which they isolated from 2 fresh placentas of rhesus monkeys in the early stages of gestation, are thought to be involved in the transfer of genetic information during embryogenesis. Although this area of investigation is in its infancy, it is likely to be quite important in the future.

IONIZING RADIATION

The effects of ionizing radiation on the development of the human fetus have been known since the early part of this century. Whether the radiation comes from a medical device or an atomic bomb, the resulting malformations are associated with the unrepaired damage of fetal cells (Merz, 1976). The character of the malformation depends on the gestational age at the time of exposure. Exposure to the 3rd week is likely to result in death of the embryo, while exposure after this time will produce abnormalities of varying severities related to the period of organogenesis at the time of exposure. At the most primitive level, x-irradiation may interfere with cell proliferation, mainly by killing the rapidly dividing embryonic cells. Cell growth may be affected and disruption of the complex patterns of neural crest migration may alter the important spatial arrangements of morphogenesis resulting in dysplasias.

PHARMACEUTICAL PREPARATIONS AND OTHER CHEMICALS

In a recent review of teratogenic agents affecting man, Smithells (1976) accepted only 5 that would be relevant to external ear development, namely thalidomide, folate antagonists, alcohol, anticonvulsants, and warfarin.

1. Alcohol. A recognizable pattern of dysmorphogenesis and dysfunction, termed the fetal alcohol syndrome, has been reported in a growing number of children whose mothers have been chronic alcoholics during pregnancy (Jones et al, 1974; Qazi and Masakawa, 1976). The variable features for this syndrome include prenatal-onset growth deficiency, microcephaly, an average IQ of 63, fine motor dysfunction, maxillary hypoplasia, short palpebral fissures, ptosis, *prominent ear crus,* heart murmur, capillary hemangiomas and various joint anomalies including dislocations, limitations and abnormal joint positions (Jones et al, 1974; Smith, 1976).

In a study by Jones et al (1974) a total of 23 alcoholic mothers were identified from a prospective study of 55,000 pregnant women and their offspring conducted by the National Institute of Neurological Diseases and Stroke. They compared these 23 women and their offspring to 56 matched controls. The frequency of perinatal mortality was 17% (4/23) for the "alcoholic" offspring and 2% (1/46) for the controls. Of the remaining 19 offspring of alcoholic women, 6 (32%) had enough abnormal features to suggest the diagnosis of fetal alcohol syndrome as compared to none in the control group. They did not provide the sex of the 6 with fetal alcohol syndrome but Qazi and Masakawa (1976) have recently reported a significant excess of females among patients with this syndrome. Although their retrospective data does not represent the sex ratio at birth, they proposed that the alcoholism in the mother may present a greater threat for survival of males than of females in the intrauterine and extrauterine milieu.

Although this data on the outcome of pregnancy for chronically alcoholic women is far from extensive and primarily retrospective, there seems little doubt that the risk of neonatal death, dysmorphogenesis and/or dysfunction to the offspring of such women is considerable. If the one small prospective study (Jones et al, 1974) is any indication, this risk is about 40%.

2. Anticonvulsants. There is little doubt now that the anticonvulsants used by epileptic mothers are teratogenic and not the disease itself. Smithells (1976), combining the data of 15 studies conducted between 1964 and 1975, found that the incidence of malformations in the offspring of epileptic mothers taking anticonvulsants was 6%. This can be compared with an incidence of 2.7% in offspring of normal controls and 1.4% in offspring of epileptic mothers not on anticonvulsants. If one calculates a contingency chi-square for the 3 groups (epileptics taking anticonvulsants; epileptics not taking anticonvulsants; controls) the observed frequencies of malformation are very significantly different from each other ($\chi_2^2 = 84.74$, $P < 0.005$). This is primarily due to the large difference between those taking anticonvulsants and controls ($\chi_1^2 = 81.95$, $P < 0.005$). The difference between epileptics not taking anticonvulsants and controls is not significant ($\chi_1^2 = 2.73$, $P > 0.05$), while the difference between the 2 epileptic groups is ($\chi_1^2 = 15.58$, $P < 0.005$).

The anticonvulsants most associated with recognizable patterns of dysmorphogenesis are phenylhydantoin (Monson et al, 1973; Hanson and Smith, 1975), trimethadione and paramethadione (German et al, 1970; Nichols, 1973; Zackai et al, 1975). Most investigators of this group of teratogens also recognize the synergistic teratogenic effect that occurs when hydantoin is combined with barbiturates, particularly phenobarbital (Fedrick, 1973; Speidel and Meadow, 1972).

The variable features of the "fetal hydantoin syndrome" include prenatal-onset growth deficiency, occasional microcephaly with mental retardation, brachycephaly, wide anterior fontanel, metopic ridging, hypertelorism, broad depressed nasal bridge, cleft lip and palate, *dysplastic ears,* low hairline, short neck, hirsutism, limb anomalies such as hypoplastic distal phalanges, small nails, digital thumb, and hip dislocation, and occasionally major cardiac malformations (Gorlin et al, 1976; Smith, 1976). The risk to the offspring of mothers taking hydantoin having the complete syndrome is approximately 10% and the risk for having some features of the disorder is an additional 33% (Hanson et al, 1976).

The variable features of the "fetal trimethadione syndrome" include prenatal-onset growth deficiency, brachycephaly, mental retardation, speech disorders, mild midface hypoplasia, upturned nose with broad and low nasal bridge, mild synophrys with eyebrow upslant, strabismus, ptosis of the eyelids, epicanthic folds, cleft lip and palate, *dysplastic ears,* micrognathia, cardiac septal defects and tetralogy of Fallot, and genital anomalies (Smith, 1976). It has been estimated by Gorlin et al (1976) that the risk to offspring of mothers taking either trimethadione or paramethadione may be as high as 65%.

The mechanism(s) of teratogenesis of these anticonvulsants are not yet understood but there may be a clue in the folate deficiency associated with phenylhydantoin and others in this drug category (Smithells, 1976).

3. Aminopterin and Methotrexate. Aminopterin and methotrexate, both folic acid antagonists, are known to be potent antineoplastic drugs. Since these agents are both toxic to rapidly dividing neoplastic cells, it is no surprise that they are also toxic to proliferating embryonic tissue. In general, aminopterin and its methyl derivative, methotrexate, have been used as abortifacients in the 1st trimester of pregnancy. The congenital malformations induced by aminopterin (Thiersch, 1952; Meltzer 1956; Warkany et al, 1959; Emerson, 1962; Shaw and Steinbach, 1968) and methotrexate (Milunsky et al, 1968; Powell and Ekert, 1971) are now well recognized.

The "aminopterin syndrome" includes prenatal-onset growth deficiency, anencephaly, hydrocephaly, microcephaly, cerebral hypoplasia, cranial bone dysplasia, synostosis of lambdoid and/or coronal sutures, maxillary hypoplasia, cleft palate, broad nasal bridge, shallow supraorbital ridges, proptosis of the eyes, *dysplastic ears,* upsweep of frontal scalp hair, mesomelia, talipes equinovarus, and hypodactyly. Of those born alive, rarely have these infants survived beyond the 1st year of life.

The "methotrexate syndrome" includes prenatal-onset growth deficiency, oxycephaly, large posterior fontanel, dysplastic frontal bone, absent coronal and lambdoidal sutures, hypertelorism, *dysplastic ears,* micrognathia, multiple anomalous ribs and absence of digits on the feet.

In a summary of reports on the use of antineoplastic agents during human pregnancy, Nishimura and Tanimura (1976) present data that indicate that the risk of dysmorphogenesis to the offspring of maternal users is at least 85% for aminopterin and 50% for methotrexate. Other apparently less teratogenic neoplastic agents include busulfan, azathioprine, and colchicine.

4. Thalidomide. The tragic story of this teratogen is well known to all and hardly needs repeating here. Excellent reviews may be found in Warkany (1971) and Nishimura and Tanimura (1976). In general, malformations of the external ear were second in frequency only to those of the limbs. They varied from preauricular tags and sinuses to severe microtia or anotia with external meatal atresia (Livingstone, 1965). In a British series of children with thalidomide-induced external ear malformations, Livingstone (1965), using polytomography, demonstrated anomalies of the middle ear ossicles in 32% of the cases.

5. Warfarin. Unlike heparin, a high molecular weight compound, coumarin derivatives such as warfarin cross the placental barrier and induce a recognized pattern of malformation termed the "fetal warfarin syndrome." Since the initial report by DiSaia (1966) at least a dozen more patients have been recognized (Hall, 1976; Sherman and Hall, 1976; Carson and Reid, 1976).

The most consistent clinical finding has been a severely hypoplastic nose. Other variable findings include intrauterine growth retardation, microcephaly with mental retardation, occipital meningomyelocele, hydrocephalus, eye anomalies, *macrotia,* stippling of the bones similar to Conradi syndrome, hypoplastic phalanges, and shortening of the limbs.

It has been thought often that the mechanism of malformation is likely to be related to decreased clotting factors and increased bleeding. Hall (1976) presents an interesting alternative based on the vitamin-K antagonist effect of warfarin. Since clotting factors, as measured in adults, are absent during the 1st trimester, and cartilage, which appears to be the most consistently affected tissue, has a poorly developed blood supply, Hall speculates that perhaps the absence of vitamin K in the growing tissue is the major problem.

This association of an unusual collection of anomalies with a rarely used medication in pregnancy is certainly more than coincidental. Thus, warfarin and related oral anticoagulants should be avoided at least during the 1st trimester of pregnancy. In mothers who require these drugs the risks should be carefully explained and alternative options carefully explored.

GENE-ENVIRONMENT INTERACTIONS

The relative contributions of the genome and environment to the variation observed in the phenotypic traits of man have long been matters of controversy. The polemics generated by such disputes have been collectively termed the "nature vs nurture argument." Although the proponents of opposing points of view have now moved away from the all-or-none positions of Galton's day and the analytic tools have become more sophisticated, such matters do not enjoy easy or readily available solutions.

The genome interacts with the environment throughout embryogenesis to form the final phenotype we observe in the newborn. Since embryogenesis has many unique developmental pathways, at each of which interaction may occur between the genome and environment, between components of the genome or between elements of the environment, we cannot really say that a particular gene or environmental agent determines a particular phenotypic outcome. Thus, we all seek to understand embryogenesis within the context of the doctrine of multifactorial association. That is, the developing fetus is the product of both its unique genetic background and the environment in which this background is forced to operate. Since the approaches to the problem have thus far been inadequate, our meager understanding of gene-environment interaction remains a constant source of frustration.

PART II
MATERIALS AND METHODS

4. The Study Design

The population base for this study consists of approximately 56,000 pregnancies and their outcomes that were studied prospectively in the Collaborative Perinatal Project (Niswander and Gordon, 1972). This study, hereafter designated NCPP, was organized and supported by the National Institute of Neurological and Communicative Disorders and Stroke (NINCDS) of the National Institutes of Health. These pregnancies were ascertained through the cooperative efforts of 14 hospitals which were affiliated with 12 universities (see Table 4-3) throughout the United States.

Women were selected for the NCPP during a 7-year period from January 2, 1959 to December 31, 1965. Initially a sampling frame, that is, those available for final selection, was established at each participating center based upon pre-established criteria. Finally, 55,908 pregnancies were registered in the NCPP population after selection from the sample frame.

The initial racial composition of the NCPP population was about 46% white, 46% black and 8% other "racial" groups, mostly Puerto Rican (Table 4-1). Approximately 5.5% of the white study pregnancies and 2.7% of the black study pregnancies were subsequently classified as "Lost to Study" cases. These were those cases for whom, for one reason or another, neither labor and delivery information nor pediatric follow-up data could be obtained. Other losses to the NCPP population included those women whose pregnancy terminated prior to 20 weeks gestation, as calculated from the first day of the gravida's last menstrual period. Ultimately there were 53,394 single births with known outcome, including 137 of unknown sex (macerated fetuses, etc) who were not utilized in calculations of singleton malformation rates (Myrianthopoulos and Chung, 1974). In addition, there were 615 twin pregnancies for whom information about the presence or absence of malformations was available. Their distribution by zygosity and completeness of pairs is listed in Table 4-2.

TABLE 4-1. "Racial" Composition of the NCPP Study Population Before Losses Due to Various Reasons*

RACIAL GROUP	NUMBER OF STUDY PREGNANCIES
White	25703
Black	25837
Puerto Rican	3795
Oriental	256
Other	317
Total	55908

*After attrition due to various reasons the racial composition of the 54009 gravidas remaining was 45% white, 47% black and 8% other "racial" groups. (All data from Niswander and Gordon, 1972 and Myrianthopoulos and Chung, 1974)

TABLE 4-2. Twin Pregnancies with Known Outcome*

ZYGOSITY	COMPLETE PAIRS	INCOMPLETE PAIRS	INDIVIDUALS
Monozygotic	187	1	375
Dizygotic	308	1	617
Zygosity unknown	87	31	205
Total	582	33	1197

*Myrianthopoulos, 1975

Since thousands of women were followed from the first months of pregnancy through labor and delivery and the children born to these NCPP mothers were followed through the 7th year of life, detailed and structured forms were developed for the study in order to provide for the collection of complete and accurate information. Procedure manuals were also developed to insure uniformity of protocol. The diagnosis of a given malformation was made in accordance with the criteria and instructions given in the appropriate manuals. These criteria were established by panels of experts to insure uniform diagnostic practices in all participating institutions.

As has been pointed out before (Myrianthopoulos and Chung, 1974), the NCPP population is ideally suited to a comprehensive investigation of congenital malformations. The prospective nature of the study insures nearly complete ascertainment and accurate assessment of the frequency of malformations in the NCPP population; the existence of prospectively collected reliable information for numerous prenatal and perinatal variables provides the opportunity to study the possible relationship of malformations to antenatal events; frequent pediatric examinations in accordance with standardized protocol over a 7-year period made possible the kind of uniform recording of observations with high accuracy that will allow future assessment of the natural history of many dysmorphic conditions.

A factor which must be considered in the interpretation of the findings of any study using this data set is that of institutional variability. Since the NCPP data have been collected at 12 institutions scattered throughout the United States, it is to be expected that they would show greater variability than if they came from a single source. As Myrianthopoulos and Chung (1974) have shown, there is indeed institutional variability in the frequency of a number of congenital malformations. A portion of this heterogeneity is, undoubtedly, real and may be due to differences in orientation and practice of medicine at each institution, as well as differences in the quality and accuracy of observations, examinations, tests and procedures. While it is not possible to estimate the extent of these differences, it is expected that they are minimal because of constant monitoring for adherence to manual instructions and to the standardized protocol.

Other possible sources of institutional heterogeneity are differences in racial composition of the sample at each institution, and geographic and other environmental differences. Institutional heterogeneity per se is not very important; however, it can be important to the extent that it influences, or is influenced by, other factors, particularly racial differences (Myrianthopoulos and Chung, 1974). Therefore, any observed institutional variability in incidence of various congenital malformations must be examined in the light of racial variability.

COMPOSITION OF THE PRESENT STUDY POPULATION

The population of the present study is composed of 2 groups, the malformed population or those children in the NCPP population with external ear and/or branchial cleft malformations, and a randomly selected group of NCPP children who were found to be without major or minor malformations.

The malformed group comprised all children (alive or deceased) who were recorded as having one or more of the following congenital malformations: preauricular sinuses, preauricular tags, anotia, microtia and other external ear malformations (cup ear, lop ear, protruding ear, etc), and branchial cleft fistulas. These patients were initially classified in the NCPP study under the following categories: 1) absence or deformity of the external auditory meatus; 2) accessory auricle; 3) preauricular skin tag; 4) deformed pinna; 5) branchial cleft anomaly. Branchial cleft anomaly in the NCPP study was defined as "preauricular sinuses and sinuses in other positions in relation to the ear." This group

58 / MATERIALS AND METHODS

essentially consisted of preauricular sinuses and branchial cleft sinuses. Another category, deformed pinna, included microtia and other lesser malformations of the external ear (cup, lop, etc). Originally there were 316 patients so designated. However, most of these cases (239) represented incompletely outfolded scapha helices, a common minor variant in the newborn, which on subsequent examinations was not present. These cases were not considered as malformations, being transient deformations at most. "Accessory auricles" proved to be a synonym for a large preauricular tag. Inclusion in the malformed group required corroboration on subsequent examinations over the 7-year follow-up period and/or a record of surgical correction. In all, 600 children were included in the malformed group.

Since the objective of this study was to test broad hypotheses, such as the hemorrhage hypothesis of Poswillo (1973), and to examine a large number of variables of unknown significance, "relative risk" analyses were considered quite suitable. Selection of an appropriate control group is undoubtedly one of the major methodologic problems encountered in the design of such analyses. Since the basic underlying assumption is that the selected "normal" group is representative of all persons without the disorder, selection bias must be avoided at all cost. The ideal procedure would have been to review and abstract the complete NCPP records of all 44,969 non-malformed children. Obviously, the time and cost of such an undertaking made this impractical. It was decided that 400 non-malformed children would be randomly selected from the non-malformed NCPP population. This represented a sample of about 1% of the total.

The number of "normals" chosen from each of the 12 centers was apportioned according to the percentage that hospital contributed to the total NCPP population, with the aid of tables of 5-digit random numbers (Guenther, 1968; Rohlf and Sokal, 1969). For each hospital the choice of table was determined randomly by the toss of a coin. The distribution of this group by hospital is given in Table 4-3. The racial distribution was 44.5% white, 48% black and 7.5% other, a distribution almost identical to the total NCPP population. The sex distribution of the children was 52% male and 48% female, again nearly identical to the 51% to 49% found in the total NCPP population.

It should be noted that in selecting the non-malformed group no a priori consideration was given to any factor that may have been suspected as having a positive association with external ear and/or branchial cleft anomalies (eg race or sex). Since when malformed and non-malformed are matched for any selected factor the influence of that factor on the disorder can no longer be studied, it was decided that matching was undesirable and that adjusting for such factors as might be matched could be handled in the statistical analysis when necessary.

TABLE 4-3. Distribution of the Non-Malformed Group by Hospital

	HOSPITAL*										
	05	10	15	31	37	45	50	55	60	66	71	82
NUMBER	87	17	19	16	30	24	23	32	24	72	30	26
PROPORTION (%)	21.7	4.3	4.7	4.0	7.5	6.0	5.7	8.0	6.0	18.0	7.5	6.5

*05: Boston Lying-in Hospital and Children's Hospital
 10: Children's Hospital of Buffalo
 15: Charity Hospital, New Orleans
 31: Columbia University
 37: Johns Hopkins Hospital
 45: Medical College of Virginia
 50: University of Minnesota
 55: New York Medical College
 60: University of Oregon
 66: Children's Hospital of Philadelphia
 71: Brown University, Providence
 82: University of Tennessee

DATA COLLECTION

The complete, original NCPP record of each patient, malformed and non-malformed, was read and abstracted on a new specially prepared data form. The criteria for the completion of the original NCPP forms can be found in the procedural manuals discussed above. There are, however, a number of points worth taking special note of here.

Two genetic data forms were employed in the NCPP study, one completed prior to the birth of the study child and one completed at the study child's 7-year pediatric examination. This provided for an update of family information, particularly for those sibs born after the proband. In addition, it often contained information about other relatives (usually 1° and/or 2°) who had a particular minor ear malformation that was not recorded on the first family history. Apparently the birth of a child with a particular external ear and/or branchial cleft malformation prompted the mothers to investigate their families and communicate this information to the history taker at the 7-year exam. This often included new information on the proband's father, sibs and grandparents. Nevertheless, information on 2° relatives other than grandparents was generally sketchy.

There are several terms which require precise definitions:

60 / MATERIALS AND METHODS

1) *Abortion:* a pregnancy terminating at less than 20 weeks gestation (excluding those which are medically induced)

2) *Birthweight:* as reported at delivery, converted from pounds and ounces to grams where necessary

3) *First Trimester:* includes the first 4 lunar months of pregnancy as calculated from the first day of the gravida's last menstrual period (LMP) as well as 1 lunar month prior to the first day of the gravida's LMP

4) *Gestation:* calculated in days between the first day of the gravida's LMP and the date of delivery — conversion to weeks was performed by dividing by seven and rounding to the nearest week

5) *Live birth:* a product of conception of 20 or more weeks gestation which at the time of complete delivery shows any sign of life, ie respiratory activity, heart beat, pulsation of cord, or definite movement of voluntary muscles

6) *Neonatal Death:* a death after birth and before 28 days

7) *Parental Age:* years completed at last birthday at the time of delivery of the study child

8) *Parity:* number of prior pregnancies exclusive of those terminating at less than 20 weeks gestation; eg parity 0 refers to a woman with no prior pregnancy of gestation 20 weeks or greater

9) *Stillbirth:* the product of conception of 20 or more weeks gestation which at the time of delivery shows no sign of life as defined under "live birth."

These terms are ones generally referred to throughout this study, both in the study forms used and in the presentation that follows. Other specific terms which if undefined may lead to ambiguity will be so defined as the need arises throughout the text.

5. Data Analysis

Since the specific aim of this study was to determine the clinical or medical import of external ear and/or branchial cleft malformations, the study was designed to answer specific questions regarding the epidemiologic, genetic, and natural historical parameters associated with these malformations. For the purpose of analysis, the methods used may be conveniently divided into epidemiologic and genetic. Naturally a number of parameters (sex of the proband, parental age, race, etc) are of value in both types of analysis and are treated as such. The description of methodologies that follows will, in general, present most analyses referred to in Part III (Results). There are, however, a few highly specialized analyses which are used in special situations and these will be described and/or referenced as they arise in presenting the results of this study.

EPIDEMIOLOGIC ANALYSIS

The method of analysis used in the present study is consistent with the classic method of epidemiologic studies (Lilienfeld, 1976). That is, many relevant factors suspected of being associated with the risk of a condition are examined one by one in relation to that condition, usually (but not always) independently of other factors.

The analysis of frequencies is generally of 2 types: 1) a test of goodness of fit of the observed frequency distribution to the expected frequency distribution representing a given a priori hypothesis; 2) a test of independence of two criteria of classification which is used to divide the frequencies into two or more classes per criteria, yielding a multicell table called the contingency table. The actual methods utilized in both types of analyses are well known and are described fully in Sokal and Rohlf (1969). In general the sample statistic used employs the chi-square (χ^2) distribution. Unless otherwise indicated, all χ^2 tests listed in the "Results" section are tests of independence, ie contingency chi-squares with the Yates correction for continuity.

62 / MATERIALS AND METHODS

In three-way tests of independence, the method of Rao (1952) was utilized. This method employs an angular transformation of the binomial proportions and then applies an analysis of variance. Corresponding to each observed proportion (p), an angle (a) is determined such that $p = \sin^2 a$. The necessary computational steps for the analysis of variance are described fully by Rao (1952) and will not be repeated here.

For continuous variables, such as age, IQ, height, etc, a t-test was used to test the hypothesis that the two sample means came from the same population. Since this test assumes that the variances in the populations from which the two samples were taken are identical, a test for homogeneity of variance was employed. The sample statistic used employs the F-distribution, with F calculated as the ratio of the greater variance over the lesser one. The computational steps for all these tests may again be found in the appropriate chapters of Sokal and Rohlf (1969).

To determine the separate effects of a series of closely related independent variables, multiple regression analyses were employed; partial correlation coefficients were obtained to measure the correlation between any pair of variables when the other specified variables have been kept constant.

Most of the suspected etiologic variables investigated in this study were discrete variables and their basic tabular presentation is the standard 2 X 2 contingency table for which a χ^2 value may be determined. It has become customary (Lilienfeld, 1976) to measure the "degree of association" between the characteristic (suspected etiologic factor) and the disease (in this case malformation) by the relative risk (RR):

$$RR = \frac{ad}{bc} = \frac{\text{Incidence of malformations in exposed group}}{\text{Incidence of malformations in nonexposed group}}$$

Lilienfeld (1976) points out that there are 2 assumptions in this RR estimate:
1) the frequency of the malformation in the population is small; 2) the malformed cases are representative of all malformed cases in the population and the non-malformed cases are representative of all non-malformed cases in the population.

The test of significance for a given RR is identical to the contingency chi-square, that is:

$$\chi^2 = \frac{(|ad-bc|-\frac{N}{2})^2 N}{(a+c)(b+d)(a+b)(c+d)} \text{, with 1 degree of freedom}$$

In addition the variance and 95% confidence limits may be calculated by the method of Haldane (1956):

$$\log_e RR = \log_e \frac{(a+1/2)(d+1/2)}{(b+1/2)(c+1/2)}$$

$$\text{Var}(\log_e RR) = \frac{1}{a+1/2} + \frac{1}{b+1/2} + \frac{1}{c+1/2} + \frac{1}{d+1/2}$$

95% confidence limits for $\log_e RR = \log_e RR \pm 1.96\left(\sqrt{\text{Var}(\log_e RR)}\,\right)$
The antilogs of these limits provide the upper and lower 95% confidence limits for the relative risk, ad/bc.

Before moving on to discuss the genetic methodologies, a number of important points should be noted:

1) An a priori significance level of 5% was set for all tests carried out in this study. We fully recognized that with multiple contingency $-\chi^2$ tests the critical significance level might be set much lower. Nevertheless, since this study was viewed as a screening procedure for possible parameters of importance that could be tested further in subsequent studies, we chose to leave the significance level at the conventional 5%.

2) Since the investigation of racial differences was of importance in this study, those variables found to be statistically significant were then further analyzed separately by race (see Chapter 8, pp 100–104).

3) Since syndromes represent an etiologically heterogeneous group of malformation complexes, it was decided a priori to exclude them from most analyses and to concentrate instead on the overwhelming majority of the cases which are nonsyndromic. Syndrome, as defined in this study, is two or more malformations in addition to the external ear and/or branchial cleft malformation(s) for which the proband was ascertained.

GENETIC ANALYSIS

The methods utilized in the genetic analysis of the malformed study population included those for both multifactorial/threshold inheritance and monogenic inheritance.

The model of multifactorial/threshold inheritance has recently been reviewed by Fraser (1976). There is assumed to be a normally distributed variable termed "liability" which is determined by a polygenic genetic predisposition and multiple environmental factors. The frequency of the disorder in the population will depend on the proportion of the population falling beyond a given threshold of liability. This threshold would be the maximum number of genetic and environmental "liability" factors one could be exposed to without subsequently displaying the abnormal phenotype at birth. Theoretically, persons falling beyond the threshold would carry more of the predisposing genes than others in the population, pushing the distribution of liability for their relatives to the right of the general population and thus resulting in more of these relatives being beyond the threshold and affected.

This model has a number of very specific predictions:
1) The risk to the relatives of probands would be some multiple of the general population frequency but considerably less than would be expected on the basis of monogenic inheritance.
2) The risk to 1° relatives is higher when the defect is more severe in the proband.
3) When one sex is affected more than the other, the recurrence risk is higher in the relatives of probands of the less frequently affected sex.
4) The recurrence risk for sibs increases with increasing numbers of affected persons in the family.
5) There is an expected increased frequency of consanguinity in the parents of probands.

Heritability (h^2) is that proportion of the total phenotypic variance that is due to additive genetic variation. An estimate of the heritability of a threshold character can be obtained from a comparison of its incidence in the general population with that in relatives of persons having the character. The computational steps used in this calculation are outlined in Emery (1976).

Segregation analysis was then used under the assumption of monogenic inheritance with some proportion of sporadic cases. On the basis of family history, the 600 malformed probands can be divided into 2 groups, familial and isolated. *Familial* is defined in this study as any other affected 1° or 2° relative. Third-degree relative data was mostly unavailable and thus could not be included in the definition. All cases not familial are termed in this study as *isolated*. Such cases are either *sporadic* which includes new mutations, phenocopies, chromosome anomalies, etc or *chance isolated,* ie those which are due to segregation at the same locus as the familial case but for one reason or another represent the only case in the family.

Since the ascertainment was through the affected children, it was *incomplete ascertainment*. If all affected children in a family are observed, but only some are probands and the others are detected through the probands, the ascertainment probability (π) is less than one. When there is frequently more than one proband per family, as is the case in a number of these families, one speaks of *multiple ascertainment*. Each family is counted as many times as there are probands (a). The maximum likelihood method of Morton (1959) was used to estimate the segregation frequency ($\emptyset$), the proportion of nonsegregating families (h), the proportion of families that give only affected children, the proportion of sporadic cases (X), and the ascertainment probability (π). As Morton (1959) points out this method is a priori in the sense of starting with a test of some null hypothesis, but a posteriori in leading by iteration to the maximum likelihood estimate if the null hypothesis is rejected. Segregation analysis was carried out separately for each racial group (blacks and whites) and for 2 parental mating types, unaffected by unaffected and affected by unaffected.

For a 2-allele locus, with genes A and a having population frequencies p and q, respectively, the Hardy-Weinberg Law predicts that after one generation of random mating with no selection, no migration and a constant rate of mutation the genotypes AA, Aa, and aa will have the frequencies p^2, $2pq$, and q^2, respectively. In the case of 2 alleles with dominance in which AA and Aa are not distinguishable from each other the gene frequencies may be estimated in the following way (Johnston, 1976):

$$p = 1-q$$

$$q = \sqrt{r/n} \text{ with a variance (Var)} = (1-q^2)/4n$$

where r = the number of persons with aa in the population; n = total population size studied. When the trait has reduced penetrance, the population frequency can be estimated as:

$$y = Z\left(\frac{\emptyset t}{\emptyset a}\right)$$

where y = the population frequency corrected for penetrance; Z = the observed population frequency of the trait; $\emptyset t$ = expected segregation frequency, 1/4 (recessive) or 1/2 (dominant); $\emptyset a$ = observed segregation frequency.

PART III
RESULTS

6. General Characteristics

There were 600 children ascertained with external ear and/or branchial cleft malformations. This is an incidence of 0.0113 (600/53,257). Of these there were 591 children with at least one ear malformation, an incidence of 0.0111, and 12 children with at least one branchial cleft malformation, an incidence of 0.0002. These 600 persons had a total of 626 external ear and/or branchial cleft malformations and these are listed along with their population frequencies in Table 6-1. Note that bilateral cases of any given malformation type were counted as one for these incidence calculations. Of those children affected, 78% were diagnosed during the neonatal period, 16% at 4 months of age and the remaining 6% by 1 year.

As detailed in Table 6-2, 42 of the 600 children presented with dysmorphic syndromes of both known and unknown etiology. We have been able to conclusively place 25 of these cases in recognized nosologic designations. The remaining 17 were either too nonspecific in their findings to be definitive or completely unknown to us. These syndromes have been listed in Table 6-2 according

TABLE 6-1. Distribution of All External Ear and Branchial Cleft Malformations

Malformation	Number	Rate per 10,000*
Preauricular sinus	446	83.74
Preauricular tags	91	17.09
Microtia	16	3.00
Other malformed pinna**	61	11.45
Branchial cleft sinus	12	2.25

*Based on a total NCPP population size of 53,257. Bilateral cases of any given malformation were counted as one for purposes of incidence calculations.

**Includes all other cases of malformed pinna. With the exception of microtia, the diagnostic labels and/or descriptions of the anomalies were not sufficiently clear to be certain of the precise nosologic category.

TABLE 6-2. Syndromic External Ear Malformation Cases in the NCPP Population

A. Syndromes of Known Etiology
  1. Pedigree syndromes
      a. *Branchio-oto-dysplasia* (autosomal dominant) with bilateral preauricular sinuses, bilateral branchial cleft sinuses and bilateral severe mixed hearing loss.
      b. *Smith-Lemli-Opitz syndrome* (autosomal recessive) with left preauricular sinus.
  2. Chromosomal syndromes
      a. *Trisomy 21* (9 cases) with microear and other pinna dysplasias.
      b. *Trisomy 18* (2 cases), one with bilateral dysplastic pinnas and one with hypoplastic lobes.
  3. Environmentally-induced syndromes
      a. *Rubella syndrome* (2 cases), one with a right preauricular sinus and the other with bilateral dysplastic pinnas.
      b. *Toxoplasmosis syndrome* with left preauricular sinus.
      c. *Amniotic band syndrome* (2 cases), one with bilateral severe pinna dysplasia and the other with right preauricular sinus; both cases had bilateral cleft lip and palate, congenital amniotic bands, and amputations of the digits.
      d. *Fetal diabetes mellitus syndrome,* with right microtia, absence of coccyx, posterior displacement of upper limbs, macerated and stillborn.
B. Syndromes of Uncertain Etiology
  1. Recurrent pattern syndromes
      a. *Abdominal muscle deficiency syndrome* with right preauricular sinus.
      b. *First and second branchial arch syndrome* (2 cases), one with right preauricular sinus and the other with bilateral preauricular tags
      c. *Holoprosencephaly* with bilateral microtia and normal chromosomes.
      d. *Prader-Willi syndrome* with bilateral lop ears.
  2. Provisionally-unique pattern syndrome
      a. *Case 1: right preauricular sinus;* bilateral isolated cleft palate; multiple hemangiomas of the face; synophrys; brachydactyly of fingers and toes; clinodactyly of 5th fingers bilaterally; abnormal separation of big toes; failure to thrive as an infant; spastic diplegia; bilateral conductive hearing loss (30-40 db); ?Klippel-Trenaunay-Weber syndrome or Sturge-Weber syndrome?
      b. *Case 2: bilateral lop ears;* hemangiomas of the nasal bridge, nape of neck and sacrum; antimongoloid obliquity of the eyes; bilateral iris colobomas; bilateral cataracts; microphthalmia; down-turned corners of the mouth; coarctation of aorta; atrial septal defect; ventricular septal defect; accessory spleen; polycystic kidneys; bicornuate uterus; hypertonic; died at 10 days of age; ?Klippel-Trenaunay-Weber syndrome or Sturge-Weber syndrome?
      c. *Case 3: left preauricular sinus;* macrocephaly; down-turned corners of the mouth; severe hypoplasia of left frontal bone; bilateral inguinal hernias; bilateral cryptorchidism; retarded locomotor development.
      d. *Case 4: bilateral preauricular sinuses;* Arnold-Chiari malformation; meningomyelocele (L3-5); microphthalmia (left>right); lumbar lordosis; right conductive hearing loss.
      e. *Case 5: bilateral lop ears with left preauricular sinus;* mitral and aortic atresia; hypoplastic left atrium, ventricle, and aortic arch; patent ductus arteriosus; patent foramen ovale; accessory spleen; acute gastric ulcers; microscrotum; bilateral cryptorchidism.
      f. *Case 6: bilateral preauricular sinuses;* exophthalmos; hypertelorism; web neck; spina bifida occulta (S-1); wide-spaced nipples; increased carrying angle; omphalocele; bilateral inguinal hernias; hypoplastic labia majora; cardiac arhythmia; normal hairline; karyotype 46,XX (no banding).

TABLE 6-2. Continued.

- g. *Case 7: right preauricular sinus;* microcephaly, bilateral exotropia; left VII nerve paresis; pectus carinatum; psychomotor retardation.
- h. *Case 8: left preauricular tag;* hydrocephalus; ventricular septal defect; patent ductus arteriosus; patent foramen ovale; aortic arch dysmorphia; hypoplastic labia majora.
- i. *Case 9: bilateral microears;* trigonocephaly; cerebellar dysfunction; antimongoloid obliquity to the eyes with left eyelid ptosis; left VII nerve palsy; short neck; low hairline; bilateral cryptorchidism; normal IQ, speech and hearing; ? 9p- or r(9)?
- j. *Case 10: bilateral poorly differentiated, protruding ears with small external auditory canals;* incomplete fusion of median and lateral nasal processes just under nares with normal vermilion border; mongoloid obliquity to the eyes; left hand postminimus; bilateral clinodactyly of the 2nd and 5th digits; normal IQ, speech and hearing.
- k. *Case 11: bilateral cryptotia;* isolated cleft palate; epicanthal folds; small orbits; short, web neck; pulmonary hypoplasia; agenesis of left diaphragm; congenital heart disease (unspecified); stenosis of ureters (hydroureters) and bilateral hydronephrosis; brachydactyly of 5th fingers with fusiform middle phalanges; right hammer toe; pes valgus; died at 44 minutes.
- l. *Case 12: bilateral dysplastic pinnas;* epicanthal folds; hypertelorism; microdontia; pyloric stenosis; bilateral 5th finger brachydactyly; mental retardation.
- m. *Case 13: bilateral microtia with meatal atresia;* large pigmented nevus above right eye; spindle-shaped hyperextensible fingers; hypoplastic thumb nails; bilateral calcaneovalgus; congenital phimosis.
- n. *Case 14: bilateral microtia;* mongoloid obliquity to the eyes; micrognathia; flattened, crooked nose; web neck; gastric hypoplasia; pulmonary hypoplasia; digital dislocations of the left hand; left knee dislocation; bilateral talipes equinovarus; died at 11 hours; history of oligohydraminios 2° to chronic leakage.
- o. *Case 15: bilateral microears;* plagiocephaly; right palpebral fissure > left; left VII nerve paresis; mental retardation; sensorineural hearing loss.
- p. *Case 16: bilateral microtia;* isolated cleft palate; hypoplastic kidneys.
- q. *Case 17: right microtia;* ventricular septal defect; absence of right thumb; 3 accessory spleens; single dysplastic kidney; absence of rectum and imperforate anus; absent urethra; tail remnant; stillborn.

C. Deformation
  Potter syndrome (1 case) with *bilateral large, flattened auricles and no extrarenal malformations.*

to the suggested classification of Cohen (1977) and have been eliminated from most further analyses for reasons enumerated previously under "Methods." Excluding syndromes, there were 549 children (0.0103) with at least one ear malformation and 11 persons (0.0002) with at least one branchial cleft malformation. There were a total of 558 children affected with 583 nonsyndromic external ear and/or branchial cleft malformations. These are listed in Table 6-3 along with their population frequencies. Again both bilateral and unilateral cases of a given malformation type were counted as one.

72 / RESULTS

TABLE 6-3. Distribution of All External Ear and Branchial Cleft Malformations Excluding Syndrome Cases

Malformation	Number	Rate per 10,000*
Preauricular sinus	431	80.93
Preauricular tags	89	16.71
Microtia	9	1.69
Other malformed pinna**	43	8.07
Branchial cleft sinus	11	2.07

*Based on a total NCPP population size of 53,257. Bilateral cases of any given malformation were counted as one for purposes of incidence calculations.

**Includes all other cases of malformed pinna. With the exception of microtia, the diagnostic labels and/or descriptions of the anomalies were not sufficiently clear to be certain of the precise nosologic category.

ETIOLOGIC RELATIONSHIPS

Since previously published cases of external ear and/or branchial cleft malformations have shown combinations of the various types in the same person or in different members of the same family, chi-square analyses were used to determine: 1) if in fact these different malformations tended to occur together more often than by chance in the same person, and 2) if they do tend to cluster, are they the result of single hits by multiple etiologies or multiple hits by single etiologies? Because there was no a priori knowledge of the etiologies of the nonsyndromic and most of the syndromic cases or their complete pleiotropic manifestations, all 600 persons were considered together for these analyses.

Table 6-4 lists the frequency of malformation "X" in cases with malformation "Y" and compares these frequencies with those of the general population without "Y." In nearly all comparisons, the probability of such clustering being random is less than 0.005.

The Poisson distribution tests the tendency of observed events to cluster. If the observations being scored occur independently, and thus are the results of single hits by multiple etiologies, then their distribution should agree with that predicted by the Poisson. Analysis of the entire study population (53,257) using standard computational methods (Sokal and Rohlf, 1969, pp. 86-87) is presented in Table 6-5. It is apparent that multiple types of anomalies in a single individual are more likely associated with multiple hits by a single etiology, and thus any given malformation of the type studied here is not necessarily etiologically distinct from any other of this type.

Based on these analyses, as well as the animal studies by Poswillo (1973) and the clinical review in chapters 1 and 3, all malformations in this study appear to share common, indistinguishable etiologies and thus are grouped together for all further analyses.

TABLE 6-4. Distribution of Malformation "X" in Cases with Malformation "Y"

"Y"	"X"	Frequency (X/Y)	Multiple of the "without 'Y' population" frequency	χ^{2}**
Preauricular sinus (446)*	Preauricular tag (7)	0.0157	9.87	43.64
	Microtia (1)	0.0022	7.89	1.01 (NS)
	Other malformed pinna (10)	0.0247	23.22	159.70
	Branchial cleft sinus (2)	0.0045	23.68	19.66
Preauricular tag (91)	Preauricular sinus (7)	0.0769	9.32	43.64
	Microtia (1)	0.0110	38.95	8.19
	Other malformed pinna (4)	0.0440	41.00	110.95
	Branchial cleft sinus (1)	0.0110	53.11	11.23
Microtia (16)	Preauricular sinus (1)	0.0625	7.48	1.01 (NS)
	Preauricular tag (1)	0.0625	36.97	8.19
Other malformed pinna (61)	Preauricular sinus (10)	0.1803	20.00	159.70
	Preauricular tag (4)	0.0656	40.09	110.95
Branchial cleft sinus (12)	Preauricular sinus (2)	0.1667	19.99	19.66
	Preauricular tag (1)	0.0833	49.30	11.23

*1. Numbers in parentheses are numbers of cases.
2. 2X2 contingency chi-square tables were constructed based on the incidence of the malformations in the general population as listed in Table 6-1. Eg 7/446 was compared to 84/52,811 in the first line of the table. Note the general population was defined in this example as all those without a preauricular sinus.

**All values less than P=0.005 with the exception of the preauricular sinus–microtia combination which was not significant (NS).

TABLE 6-5. Observed and Expected Distribution of External Ear and/or Branchial Cleft Malformations

Number of anomaly types per proband[a]	Total number		Deviation from Expected[d]
	Observed[b]	Expected[c]	
0	52,657	52,637.5	+
1	574	615.9	−
2	26	3.6	+

[a] Eg a proband with a preauricular sinus and a preauricular tag whether on the same side or not, was considered to have 2 anomaly types, while a proband with bilateral preauricular sinuses was considered to have 1 anomaly type.

[b] Total number in NCPP study = 53,257
Total number of considered malformations = 626
Mean number of considered malformations per NCPP study child = 0.0118
Total number of NCPP study children with considered malformations = 600

[c] Calculated from Poisson distribution (Sokal and Rohlf, 1969, pp. 86-87)

[d] Goodness of fit χ^2 = 142.24 ($P < 0.005$)

TABLE 6-6. Distribution of Nonsyndromic Malformations: Familial vs Isolated

Malformation	Familial*	Isolated*
Preauricular sinus	27 (6.26)	404 (93.74)
Preauricular tags	6 (6.74)	83 (93.26)
Microtia	0 (0.00)	9 (100.00)
Other malformed pinna	7 (16.28)	36 (83.72)
Branchial cleft sinus	0 (0.00)	11 (100.00)
Total number	40 (6.86)	543 (93.14)
Percent of total NCPP study population (53,257)	0.08	1.01

*Numbers in parentheses are the frequencies in percent of familial and isolated in each malformation category.

FAMILIAL vs ISOLATED

The terms familial and isolated are used here as defined in "Methods." An "affected 1° or 2° relative" is now defined as one with any external ear and/or branchial cleft malformation, regardless of whether it is identical to that in the proband or not. The distribution of all malformed cases according to the desig-

TABLE 6-7. Laterality of Malformations in Nonsyndromic Cases

	Bilateral	Unilateral =	Right +	Left +	Unspecified
Familial	16	19	11	7	1
Isolated	150	373	202	166	5
$2 \times 2 \chi^2$		3.78*	0.08		
Combined	166	392	213	173	6

*$P \approx 0.05$

nations "familial" or "isolated" and the distribution according to malformation type can be seen in Table 6-6. The proportion of isolated cases was greater than 80% in all malformation categories.

LATERALITY

The analysis of malformation laterality is presented in Table 6-7. It appears that the tendency to be bilateral or unilateral may be dependent on the case type, familial or isolated ($\chi^2 = 3.78$, $P \approx 0.05$). The frequency of bilateral cases is considerably higher among familial cases (0.46) and, conversely, the frequency of unilateral cases is higher among isolated cases (0.71). The unilateral distribution, right vs left, was independent of case type (familial or isolated). However, there was a significant predilection for the right side ($\chi_1^2 = 40.32$; $P < 0.005$) if one takes the null hypothesis to be an equal distribution on both sides.

ADDITIONAL MALFORMATIONS IN THE NONSYNDROMIC CASES

Although we have already eliminated syndromes (2+ malformations in addition to the one being studied) from the analyses, there exists a group of patients in which a single additional malformation, major or minor, can be seen. Such events may represent a chance occurrence or a real association in which the occurrence of the two malformations happens with greater frequency than reasonably can be expected by chance alone. The pros and cons of whether these statistically significant associations can be classified as syndromes in their own right will be discussed later.

Table 6-8 shows that the frequency of a single additional malformation in the nonsyndromic cases was significantly greater ($\chi_1^2 = 103.51$; $P < 0.005$) than the malformation frequency in the remaining NCPP population. On closer inspection we can see that this frequency was significantly higher in the isolated cases but not so in the familial cases. For this reason the association of a particular malformation with an external ear and/or branchial cleft malformation is considered separately for familial and isolated probands (Table 6-9).

76 / RESULTS

TABLE 6-8. The Frequency of a Single Additional Malformation in the Nonsyndromic Cases

Case type	Malformation type*			Combined vs combined (case type vs NCPP)
	Major	Minor	Combined	
Familial	2/35 (0.06)	6/35 (0.17)	8/35 (0.23)	$\chi^2 = 0.98$
Isolated	75/523 (0.14)	91/523 (0.17)	166/523 (0.32)	$\chi^2 = 104.05**$
Combined	77/558 (0.14)	97/558 (0.17)	174/558 (0.31)	$\chi^2 = 103.51**$
Remaining NCPP population	---	---	8,114/52,699 (0.15)	---

*The numerator is the number of malformed, the denominator is the total number of cases for each case type and the number in parentheses is the frequency which may be converted to percent by multiplying by 100.
**$P < 0.005$

TABLE 6-9. Congenital Malformations at Age 1 Year with Frequencies Significantly Greater ($P < 0.05$) in Isolated Nonsyndromic Cases Than in Remaining NCPP Population at Age 1 Year

Malformation*	Rate per 10,000		$2 \times 2 \chi^2$
Major	Proband group	NCPP group	
1. Craniosynostosis (4)	76.5	4.6	38.22
2. Kyphoscoliosis (3)	57.4	6.8	11.83
3. Pectus carinatum (2)	38.2	2.5	12.54
4. Congenital heart disease (12)	229.4	74.1	14.63
5. Inguinal hernia (13)	248.5	133.3	4.35
6. Dysmorphic ureters (2)**	38.2	0.9	30.10
Minor			
1. Digital dysmorphia, mild (4)***	76.5	9.9	16.00
2. Strawberry/port wine hemangioma (21)	401.5	225.9	6.42
3. Pigmented nevus (8)	153.0	45.3	10.77
4. Café-au-lait spots (31)	592.7	70.0	182.92
5. Vitiligo (2)	38.2	0.0	112.69

*There are 523 nonsyndromic isolated proband cases and the number in parentheses indicates how many of these had a particular malformation.
**Includes atretic and/or double ureters.
***Includes such anomalies as mildly hypoplastic distal phalanges, notched distal phalanges, etc.

In an attempt to avoid spurious associations, only those malformations which occurred 2 or more times in the proband population were considered for analysis. For isolated probands, 22 such malformation frequencies were analyzed, of which 11 were significant at the 5% level or less. On the basis of chance alone we

TABLE 6-10. Sex Ratios of Nonsyndromic Proband Sibships

Group	Status	Male	Female	Total	M/F ratio
Familial	Probands	18	17	35	1.06
	Affected sibs	9	15	24	0.60
	Unaffected sibs	57	34	91	1.68*
	Total	84	66	150	1.27
Isolated	Probands	275	248	523	1.11
	Unaffected sibs	554	581	1135	0.95
	Total	829	829	1658	1.00
Combined	Probands	293	265	558	1.11
	Affected sibs	9	15	24	0.60
	Unaffected sibs	611	615	1226	0.99
	Total	913	895	1,808	1.02

*Significantly different from the 1.04 (.51/.49) M/F Ratio found in the NCPP population and other study populations of large size ($\chi_1^2 = 4.93$; $P < 0.05$).

would have expected only 1 to be significant. The significantly associated malformations are listed in Table 6-9. In addition there were a number of malformations which could not be analyzed because of a lack of NCPP population frequencies. These included 2 cases of neonatal teeth, 2 of ankyloglossia, 2 of eyelid ptosis, and 4 of severe myopia.

Among the familial cases there was only one malformation that occurred more than once, lacrimal duct stenosis (2 cases). The frequency of this malformation was significantly higher than the remaining NCPP population ($\chi_1^2 = 47.73$; $P < 0.005$). This contrasts with the isolated cases in which there were also 2 cases but the frequency was not significantly different from the remaining NCPP population ($\chi_1^2 = 1.09$; $P > 0.1$).

SEX RATIOS

The male/female sex ratio (Table 6-10) was 1.06 for familial probands, 1.11 for isolated probands and 1.11 overall. None of these ratios was significantly different from the 1.04 ratio found in the overall NCPP population and other study populations of large size.

From Table 6-10 one can see that the overall male to female sex ratio in the familial sibships is not significantly different from 1.04. However, after partitioning

TABLE 6-11. Racial Distribution of the Nonsyndromic Cases*

Case type**		Black		White		Other	Total	
Familial	Malformed	27 (0.11)		6 (0.03)		2 (0.05)	35	53,
	Remainder	25,099		24,147		3,976	53,222	
	2 X 2 χ^2		11.36***		0.14			
Isolated	Malformed	405 (1.61)		95 (0.39)		23 (0.58)	523	53,
	Remainder	24,721		24,058		3,955	52,734	
	2 X 2 χ^2		180.86***		2.37			
Combined	Malformed	432 (1.72)		101 (0.42)		25 (0.63)	558	53,
	Remainder	24,694		24,052		3,953	52,699	
	2 X 2 χ^2		193.66***		2.93			

*Numbers in parentheses are malformed frequencies in percent.
**Racial type and case type (familial, etc) were independent of one another (χ_2^2 = 0.146, P > 0.9).
***P < 0.005

the data into affected and unaffected sibs, these data show that there is a significant excess of unaffected males ($\chi_1^2 = 4.93$; P < 0.05) which complements the slight excess of affected female sibs. By contrast, there were no significant deviations from expected in the isolated sibships when they were analyzed in this way.

RACE

The frequency of external ear and/or branchial cleft malformations was more than 4 times greater in blacks than in whites and this was highly significant (Table 6-11). It should be noted that the race of the proband was independent of whether the proband was a familial or isolated case ($\chi_2^2 = 0.46$; P > 0.9). Table 6-12 shows that the differences between the races is accounted for by the highly significant excess of preauricular sinuses among blacks. It should be noted, however, that the frequency of cases in which a proband had two or more different types of external ear and/or branchial cleft malformations is about 4% in both whites (4/101) and blacks (19/432) and thus the phenomenon of a given etiology being associated with more than one type of ear malformation in a single individual is evident in both races.

INSTITUTION

Table 6-13 shows that the overall frequency of malformed persons was highly dependent on the institution studied ($\chi_{11}^{21} = 793.19$; P > 0.005). In addition, the frequency of familial or isolated malformations was also highly dependent on insti-

TABLE 6-12. Distribution of Nonsyndromic Malformations by Race and Phenotype

Malformation	Whites		Blacks	
	Number	Rate per 10,000*	Number	Rate per 10,000*
Preauricular sinus	43	17.80	374	148.85***
Preauricular tag	33	13.66	48	19.10 (NS)
Microtia	4	1.66	5	1.99 (NS)
Other malformed pinna**	20	8.28	18	7.16 (NS)
Branchial cleft sinus	5	2.07	6	2.39 (NS)

*Based on a total NCPP white population of 24,153 and NCPP black population of 25,126. Bilateral cases of any given malformation were counted as one for purposes of incidence calculations.
**Includes all other cases of malformed pinna. With the exception of microtia, the diagnostic labels and/or descriptions of the anomalies were not sufficiently clear to be certain of the precise nosologic category.
***Significantly greater than the incidence in whites (χ_1^2 = 250.48, P < 0.005)
(NS) — no significant difference between the races

tution, the χ_{11}^2 being 35.43 (P < 0.005) and 790.01 (P < 0.005), respectively. However, the proportion of familial to isolated cases was not quite as variable among institutions (χ_{11}^2 =25.00; P < 0.01). The incidence of familial cases tended to follow the overall incidence of ear malformation cases in magnitude, hospital by hospital.

RACIAL AND INSTITUTIONAL VARIABILITY

Upon further inspection of Table 6-13, one finds that there is considerable variation in racial composition among hospitals (χ_{11}^2 = 29147.73; P < 0.005), in addition to the significant variation in malformation frequency among hospitals and races already noted above. The problem arises as to whether the racial variation in malformation frequency is the same in all hospitals. That is, we had to determine whether there is interaction between race and institution. To do this we employed first an angular transformation of the binomial proportions and then applied an analysis of variance (Rao, 1952). The results of this analysis are presented in Table 6-14.

As expected the overall race differences were highly significant (χ_1^2 =47.04; P < 0.005). This was even more so (χ_1^2 = 133.25; P < 0.005) when racial variation was considered after eliminating the institutional differences. Similarly institutional variation, after eliminating racial differences, was also highly significant (χ_{10}^2 = 297.31; P < 0.005). However, the interaction χ^2 was not significant, indicating that

TABLE 6-13. Distribution of Nonsyndromic Malformed Persons by Institution

	Hospital*												
	05	10	15	31	37	45	50	55	60	66	71	82	Total
Malformed-Familial (F)	6	0	4	2	1	4	0	4	7	0	1	6	35
Malformed-Isolated (I)	57	3	60	35	17	38	12	25	26	58	14	178	523
Total Malformed (M)	63	3	64	37	18	42	12	29	33	58	15	184	558
Total Normal (N)	11,540	2,322	2,458	2,055	3,996	3,225	3,080	4,298	3,175	9,484	3,932	3,271	52,836**
M/M+Nx100	0.54	0.13	2.54	1.77	0.45	1.29	0.39	0.67	1.03	0.61	0.38	5.33	1.05
F/M+Nx100	0.05	0.00	0.16	0.10	0.03	0.12	0.00	0.09	0.22	0.00	0.03	0.18	0.07
I/M+Nx100	0.49	0.13	2.38	1.67	0.42	1.17	0.39	0.58	0.81	0.61	0.35	5.16	0.98
F/Mx100	9.52	0.00	6.25	5.40	5.56	9.52	0.00	13.79	21.21	0.00	6.67	3.26	6.27
I/Mx100	90.48	100.00	93.75	94.60	94.44	90.48	100.00	86.21	78.79	100.00	93.33	96.74	93.73
Number of:													
Whites	10,282	2,244	0	617	879	814	2,934	258	2,274	855	3027	21	24,205
Blacks	1,135	55	2,522	857	3,128	2,447	18	1,508	859	8,363	858	3,434	25,184
Others	186	26	0	618	7	6	140	2561	75	324	62	0	4,005

*See Table 4-3
**Includes 137 individuals of unknown sex (Myrianthopoulos and Chung, 1974).

TABLE 6-14. Racial and Institutional Variability

		Hospital												
		05	10	15	31	37	45	50	55	60	66	71	82	Total
Whites	Affected	46	3	0	4	0	2	12	1	19	2	11	1	101
	Total	10,282	2,244	0	617	879	814	2,934	258	2,274	855	3,027	21	24,205
Blacks	Affected	16	0	64	27	18	40	0	10	14	56	4	183	432
	Total	1,135	55	2,522	857	3,128	2,447	18	1,508	859	8,363	858	3,434	25,184

Analysis of χ^2*

	Degrees of freedom	χ^2
Race	1	47.04**
Institution	10	297.31**
Interaction	10	16.57NS
TOTAL***	21	447.13**

*Since there were no whites in the population of Hospital 15, this hospital was not considered in the analysis.
**$P < 0.005$; NS = not significant
***Note that the various components of χ^2 do not add up to the total because the proportions are based on different numbers (Rao, 1952).

82 / RESULTS

the racial variation in malformation frequency was independent of the institutional variation. Nevertheless, although the racial variation was quite real, there remained considerable institutional differences after racial variation was eliminated.

A more precise visualization of this institutional heterogeneity can be gotten by dividing the mean institutional χ^2 by the mean interaction χ^2. In this case, this variance ratio ($F_{10,10} = 17.94$) is highly significant ($P < 0.001$).

7. Genetics

It has already been demonstrated that there are highly significant racial differences in the incidence of external ear and/or branchial cleft malformations. These differences may reflect important genetic differences between blacks and whites. For this reason it was decided to analyze the racial groups separately.

Since there was relatively little evidence for a familial aggregation of affected individuals (Table 6-6), it was apparent that most cases were not likely to be inherited in a simple mendelian fashion. Rather than entertain elaborate etiologic explanations, it was felt appropriate to investigate initially the suitability of the classic multifactorial/threshold model which includes as one of its features polygenic inheritance. The predictions of this model have been described in Chapter 5.

Examination of the frequency of these malformations in the 1° relatives of probands reveals that there is a 3.3-fold increase in the incidence among white 1° relatives and virtually no increase among black 1° relatives (Table 7-1). Utilizing the most conservative predictions, $p^{.6}$ in whites and $p^{.8}$ in blacks (Czeizel and Tusnady, 1972), for calculating the respective expected incidences of a polygenically determined trait in the 1° relatives of white and black probands, the observed number of affected 1° relatives in both races differed significantly from the expected; the χ^2 in whites was 6.49 ($P < 0.025$) and in blacks 23.12 ($P < 0.005$).

TABLE 7-1. The Incidence of External Ear and/or Branchial Cleft Malformations in the First-Degree Relatives of Probands

	WHITES			BLACKS		
	Affected	Unaffected	Frequency	Affected	Unaffected	Frequency
General population	101	24153	0.0042	432	25126	0.0172
Observed 1° relatives	6	426	0.0139	32	1816	0.0173
Expected 1° relatives*	16	416	0.0370	72	1776	0.0390

*Based upon an expected frequency of $p^{.6}$ in whites and $p^{.8}$ in blacks, where p is the general population frequency in each race. The exponent for p is estimated from tables provided by Czeizel and Tusnady (1972).

Again employing predictions of the model, the severity of the defect should be proportional to the number of genetic and/or environmental liability factors present in the affected individual. Theoretically, the relatives of more severely affected probands should be at greater risk to express the phenotype. As can be seen in Table 7-2 this was not true for either whites ($\chi_1^2 = 0.19; P > 0.5$) or blacks ($\chi_1^2 = 0.018; P > 0.5$). Furthermore, holding the number of children born after the proband constant by regression (Table 7-3), only 0.06% in blacks and virtually 0.00% in whites of the total variation in the number of children affected after the proband could be accounted for by the variation of the number affected up to and including the proband. Neither of the partial correlations associated with this prediction of the model was significantly different from 0. Even when the number of children born after the proband was allowed to vary freely, the number of children affected up to and including the proband could only account for 0.05% of the variation in risk to black sibs born subsequent to the proband and virtually 0.00% of this same variation in whites. Finally there was no consanguinity in any of the families studied.

TABLE 7-2. Proband Severity and the Malformation Risk to First-Degree Relatives

Proband Severity Group	WHITE 1° RELATIVES			BLACK 1° RELATIVES		
	Affected	Unaffected	Frequency	Affected	Unaffected	Frequency
Microtia	0	20	0.0000	0	24	0.0000
Other	6	406	0.0146	32	1792	0.0175

TABLE 7-3. The Risk to Sibs Born After the Proband with Increasing Numbers of Affected Sibs in the Proband Sibship

Partial Correlations*	WHITES		BLACKS	
	Partial Coefficient (r)	Coefficient of Determination (r^2)	Partial Coefficient (r)	Coefficient of Determination (r^2)
$X_1 X_2 . Y$	−0.122878	0.015099	0.018029	0.000325
$X_1 Y . X_2$	0.000000	0.000000	−0.024832	0.000617
$X_2 Y . X_1$	0.000000	0.000000	0.211926**	0.044913

*X_1 = number of affected sibs up to and including the proband
 X_2 = number of sibs born after the proband
 Y = number of sibs affected after the proband
**P < 0.001

Heritability (h^2) estimates were calculated for each race from the population and observed 1° data presented in Table 7-1. For whites h^2 in percent was 29.59 ± 11.02 and for blacks 0.16 ± 5.93. It should be noted that since these estimates are in large measure based on sib data, the values for both races are probably inflated unless one is willing to assume that the dominance component of the genetic variance is equal to 0, an assumption which is most likely untenable in the case of sibs. For this reason these estimates may be a closer approximation to a measure of the relative genetic determination of the malformations, ie a measure of that portion of the total phenotypic variance which is genetic and not just the additive component of that genetic variance. Unfortunately, there was not sufficient parent-offspring or reliable enough 2° data to make better estimates of the heritability. In any case, it would appear that the degree of environmental determination in both races is considerable, strikingly so in blacks.

In summary, thus far, the data analysis has demonstrated: 1) the incidences in the 1° relatives of probands do not conform with the predicted incidences of a multifactorial/threshold (including polygenic) trait; 2) the severity of the proband's malformation and/or the number of affected up to and including the proband has no apparent relationship to the risk of recurrence in future sibs; 3) the heritability estimates are low in both races, particularly so in blacks. Thus, the classic multifactorial/threshold model which includes polygenic inheritance is not satisfactory in explaining these data. Consequently, it became necessary to search for alternative explanations.

SEGREGATION ANALYSIS

The frequency of familial probands among all probands was 6% in both races. As noted in the last chapter, there are a number of parameters which distinguish the familial group of probands from the isolated. These include: 1) the frequency of bilateral cases is considerably greater in the familial group; 2) an increased frequency of single additional malformations of many types in the isolated cases only; 3) in the familial group only, a slight excess of affected females which is complemented by a significant excess of unaffected males. These dichotomies and the fact that the pedigrees of about 1/2 of the familial probands demonstrated vertical transmission through 2 and 3 generations made it reasonable to regard at least these probands as likely monogenic cases and to estimate the proportions of sporadic and familial cases among the total population of isolated cases as well as the segregation frequency of the familial cases. This was accomplished by the method outlined by Morton (1959) which employs maximum likelihood scores.

Regarding blacks, the largest group of affected persons, the distribution of unaffected by unaffected (U X U) matings by sibship size and number of affected children is found in Table 7-4. Initially assuming that all multiplex sibships were familial and the remaining isolated (simplex) sibships were truly sporadic, first estimates (Table

86 / RESULTS

TABLE 7-4. Distribution of Black Sibships of Unaffected × Unaffected (U × U) Matings by Sibship Size and Number of Affected Children

Number of Affected Children	SIBSHIP SIZE												
	1	2	3	4	5	6	7	8	9	10	11	12	15	TOTAL
1	111	73	78	58	27	21	15	8	4	3	2	3	1	404
2	–	1	2	2	0	1	1	0	0	0	0	1	0	8
3	–	–	0	0	0	0	1	0	0	0	0	0	0	1
TOTAL	111	74	80	60	27	22	17	8	4	3	2	4	1	413

TABLE 7-5. Initial Estimates of $\emptyset$ and Π for Black Multiplex Sibships of Unaffected × Unaffected Matings Grouped by Sibship Size

s	n_s	r_s	a_s	a(s-1)	a(r-1)	a(a-1)
12	1	2	2	22	2	2
7	2	5	2	12	3	0
6	1	2	2	10	2	2
4	2	4	3	9	3	2
3	2	4	4	8	4	4
2	1	2	2	2	2	2
TOTAL	9	19	15	63	16	12

a) s = sibship size; n_s = number of sibships of size s;
r = number of affecteds in sibships of size s;
a = number of probands in sibships of size s

b) $\hat{\emptyset} = \dfrac{\Sigma a (r-1)}{\Sigma a (s-1)} = \dfrac{16}{63} = 0.254$

$\hat{\Pi} = \dfrac{\Sigma a (a-1)}{\Sigma a (r-1)} = \dfrac{12}{16} = 0.750$

7-5) of the segregation frequency ($\emptyset$) and ascertainment probability (Π) were 0.254 and 0.750, respectively, as calculated by the Weinberg Proband Method (Crow, 1965). Iteration by SEGRAN (Morton, 1959) and utilizing all U × U matings revealed the best estimates to be $\emptyset = 0.096 \pm 0.036$, X = 0.804 ± 0.062, and $\Pi = 0.750 \pm 0.104$. The results would indicate that there are a substantial number of isolated cases which are in fact chance isolated and not sporadic. Since there is no evidence that there are

TABLE 7-6. Probability (Q) in Blacks that an Isolated Case is Sporadic Given an U X U Mating With a Negative Family History for Various Family Sizes of S Children

S	1	2	3	4	5	6	7	8	9	10
Q*	0.804	0.819	0.834	0.847	0.860	0.872	0.883	0.893	0.902	0.911

*$Q = \dfrac{X}{X \pm (1-X)(1-\emptyset)^{S-1}}$ (Chung and Brown, 1970), where X = proportion of sporadic cases and $\emptyset$ = segregation frequency

TABLE 7-7. Distribution of Black Sibships of Affected X Unaffected (A X U) Matings by Sibship Size and Number of Affected Children

Number of Affected Children	SIBSHIP SIZE						
	1	2	3	4	5	8	TOTAL
1	2	2	1	1	2	0	8
2	-	1	0	0	0	1	2
TOTAL	2	3	1	1	2	1	10

affected relatives in either parental line for these sibships, one may then use the method of Chung and Brown (1970) to estimate the probability (Q) that an isolated case with 2 unaffected parents is sporadic. These are listed for various sibship sizes in Table 7-6 and may be utilized in counseling.

The distribution of affected by unaffected (A X U) black matings by sibship size and number of affected children is found in Table 7-7. Since the number of affected children and the number of probands was the same, Π was taken to be equal to 1. This allowed us to test the null hypothesis that $\emptyset = 0.5$ and to arrive at a first maximum likelihood estimate of the observed $\emptyset$ using the method described by Elandt-Johnson (1971). It should be noted that although there is vertical (as well as male-to-male) transmission in these families the null hypothesis, $\emptyset = 0.5$, is compatible with either autosomal dominant inheritance of a rare mutant or autosomal recessive inheritance of a common mutant in which a substantial number of Aa X aa matings are to be found. The results of this initial analysis are presented in Table 7-8. The null hypothesis, $\emptyset = 0.5$, was rejected ($Z = 8.16$, $P < 0.005$) and the first estimate of $\emptyset$ was calculated as 0.209 ± 0.102. We were unable to reject the hypothesis that these

TABLE 7-8. Black Sibships of Affected X Unaffected Matings: Testing $H_0: \emptyset=0.5$ and Calculations for First Maximum Likelihood Estimate of $\emptyset$

			Affected Children			
			Obs.	Exp.		Z^2 with
S	n_s	Sn_s	r_s	$n_s A_s$*	$n_s B_s$*	1 d.f.
2	3	6	4	3.999	0.666	0.000
3	1	3	1	1.714	0.490	1.040
4	1	4	1	2.133	0.782	1.641
5	2	10	2	5.162	2.164	4.620
8	1	8	2	4.016	1.945	2.090
TOTAL	8	31	10(R)	17.024	6.047	9.391 = Z^2 TOTAL, 5d.f.

*Computed from tables provided by Elandt-Johnson (1971)

a) Test of $H_0: \emptyset = 0.5$

$$Z^2_{\substack{comb. \\ 1 d.f.}} = \frac{(R - \sum_{s=1}^{\tilde{s}} n_s A_s)^2}{\sum_{s=1}^{s} n_s B_s} = \frac{(10-17.024)^2}{6.047} = 8.16, P < 0.005$$

b) Homogeneity of data set

$$Z^2 \text{ diff} = Z^2 \text{ TOTAL} - Z^2 \text{ comb.} = 1.23, P > 0.5$$
$$\quad\quad 4 d.f. \quad\quad 5 d.f. \quad\quad 1 d.f.$$

c) $\emptyset_1 = \emptyset_0 + U(\emptyset_0)/I(\emptyset_0) =$ First estimate $\emptyset$

$$U(\emptyset_0) = \frac{1}{\emptyset_0(1-\emptyset_0)} (R - \sum_{s=1}^{s} n_s A_s)$$

$$I(\emptyset_0) = \frac{1}{\emptyset_0^2 (1-\emptyset_0)^2} \sum_{s=1}^{S} n_s B_s$$

$$Var(\emptyset) = 1/I(\emptyset_0)$$

$$\therefore \emptyset = 0.209 \pm 0.102$$

family data are homogeneous ($Z^2_4 = 1.23, P > 0.50$). Iteration of these A X U data by SEGRAN (Morton, 1959) with $\emptyset = 0.25$ as the initial estimate revealed the best estimates to be $\emptyset = 0.132 \pm 0.082$, $\Pi = 1.00 \pm 0.23$, and $X = -0.162 \pm 0.494$.

Regarding whites, the distribution of unaffected by unaffected (U X U) matings by sibship size and number of affected children is found in Table 7-9. Since there

TABLE 7-9. Distribution of White Sibships of Unaffected X Unaffected (U X U) Matings by Sibship Size and Number of Affected Children

Number of Affected Children	SIBSHIP SIZE								
	1	2	3	4	5	6	7	8	TOTAL
1	19	18	21	15	11	6	5	1	96
2	–	0	1	1	0	0	0	0	2
TOTAL	19	18	22	16	11	6	5	1	98

TABLE 7-10. Probability (Q) in Whites that an Isolated Case is Sporadic Given an U X U Mating With a Negative Family History for Various Family Sizes of S Children

S	1	2	3	4	5	6	7	8	9	10
Q*	0.828	0.843	0.856	0.869	0.881	0.891	0.901	0.910	0.919	0.926

$$*Q = \frac{X}{X + (1-X)(1-\emptyset)^{S-1}}$$ (Chung and Brown, 1970), where X = proportion of sporadic cases and $\emptyset$ = segregation frequency

were only 2 multiplex U X U families, first estimates were not calculated from these data but were taken to be those calculated for blacks, ie $\emptyset = 0.25$, $\Pi = 0.75$, and $X = 0.90$. Iteration with SEGRAN (Morton, 1959) on the total U X U data yielded as best estimates $\emptyset = 0.101 \pm 0.079$, $X = 0.828 \pm 0.118$, and $\Pi = 0.358 \pm 0.231$. Again, since there was no evidence that there were affected relatives in either parental line for these white U X U sibships, one may use the method of Chung and Brown (1970) to estimate the probability (Q) that an isolated case is sporadic (Table 7-10).

Unfortunately only 3 A X U parental matings were found in the population of white probands. These are too few to provide meaningful conclusions. Nevertheless it is worth noting that a simple Weinberg Proband Method calculation gave a segregation estimate of $\emptyset = 0.14$, consistent with the results in other race-mating type groups.

Based on the results of the total segregation analysis, there are at least 2 independent sets of assumptions one may use to estimate the gene frequencies in each race. The first set (A_1) is as follows: a) that portion of the affected cases which is nonsporadic is genetic in origin; b) single locus, two alleles; c) trait behaves as a mendelian recessive, ie $\emptyset_t = 0.25$, with reduced penetrance; d) the homologous allele ("normal") behaves as a dominant and heterozygotes are phenotypically indistinguishable from homozygotes; e) Hardy-Weinberg equilibrium. The second set (A_2) differs in that the

90 / RESULTS

TABLE 7-11. Gene Frequency Estimates by Race Under Condition Set A_1

	WHITES	BLACKS
p	0.955 ± 0.003	0.903 ± 0.003
q	0.045 ± 0.003	0.097 ± 0.003
p^2	0.912	0.816
2pq	0.086	0.175
q^2	0.002	0.009

$$y = \frac{(1-x)(UU) + AU}{N}$$

$$q = \sqrt{y\left(\frac{\emptyset_t}{\emptyset_a}\right)}$$

$$p = 1 - q$$

$$Var = \frac{(1-q^2)}{4N}$$

y = the observed population frequency of the *genetic* trait

x = proportion of cases that are sporadic

UU = number of proband cases from normal x normal matings

AU = number of proband cases from affected x normal matings

N = total population size studied

$\emptyset_t$ = theoretic segregation value

$\emptyset_a$ = observed segregation frequency

p = frequency of the normal dominant allele

q = frequency of the mutant recessive allele

trait behaves as a mendelian dominant ($\emptyset_t = 0.5$) with reduced penetrance but again the homozygotes and heterozygotes are phenotypically indistinguishable; the "normal" allele behaves as a recessive. Calculations of gene frequencies and their standard errors for each race under each set of assumptions can be found in Tables 7-11 and 7-12.

It would appear from these calculations (Tables 7-11 and 7-12) that we are given the choice between a common recessive trait with about 40% penetrance or a "rare" dominant trait with about 20% penetrance, assuming one accepts the nonsporadic cases as being mendelian in character. One note of caution—these figures, of course, represent only crude estimates and include many hidden assumptions such as random mating, no selection, and, perhaps the most troublesome of all, that all sporadic cases are nongenetic. In addition, given the relatively low value of Π in the white population (0.36), the gene frequencies for this racial group may be a considerable underestimate.

TABLE 7-12. Gene Frequency Estimates by Race Under Condition Set A_2

	WHITES	BLACKS
p	0.0021 ± 0.0002	0.0094 ± 0.0004
q	0.9979 ± 0.0002	0.9906 ± 0.0004
p^2	0.000004	0.000089
2pq	0.004066	0.018680
q^2	0.995930	0.981231

$$y = \frac{(1-x)(UU) + AU}{N}$$

$$q = \sqrt{1 - y\left(\frac{\phi_t}{\phi_a}\right)}$$

$$p = 1 - q$$

$$Var = \frac{(1-q^2)}{4N}$$

p = frequency of the mutant dominant allele
q = frequency of the normal recessive allele

PARENTAL AGE, MUTATION AND THE SPORADIC CASES

Penrose (1955) pointed out that the difference between mean birth ages of fathers and mothers (p-m) for a particular trait is a sensitive measure of gene mutation. If both means are increased but the differences remain small, the trait is likely due to long exposure to natural background radiation; if the mean paternal age is increased relative to maternal age and the differences are large, the trait is likely due to gene copy failure during spermatogenesis; if the mean maternal age is increased relative to paternal age and the differences are large, the trait is likely due to long exposure to chemical mutagens. Evidence for any of these possibilities was specifically searched for in the isolated cases which include a large proportion of sporadic cases.

Table 7-13 lists the observed parental age means and differences for the isolated malformed and non-malformed groups. The difference (p-m) in the isolated malformed group is 10 months greater than in the non-malformed group and this difference is significant ($t_{912} = 2.6693$; $P < 0.01$). However, the results are not that

TABLE 7-13. Parental Age, Mutation and Isolated Cases

Group	Mean Age		Difference	Estimated Mean Age for Mutants**	
	Maternal (m)*	Paternal (p)	(p-m)*	Maternal	Paternal
Isolated	23.53 ± 5.96	27.49 ± 7.64	3.96	26.07	29.53
Control	24.49 ± 6.22	27.63 ± 7.26	3.14	—	--

*significant difference between groups $P < 0.01$
**$m_1 = m_0 + (v/m_0)$ where m_0 and v = mean maternal age and variance of the general population
m_1 = expected mean maternal age for mutants
$p_1 = p_0 + (v/p_0)$ where p_0 and   v = mean paternal age and variance of the general population
p_1 = expected mean paternal age for mutants
(Derivations of these equations may be found in Cavalli-Sforza and Bodmer, 1971, pp. 114-115.)

TABLE 7-14. Parental Age and Parity: Regression Analysis

Partial Correlations	Partial Coefficients**
1Y·2345	0.0637
2Y·1345	-0.0575
3Y·1245	-0.0191
4Y·1235	-0.0039
5Y·1234	-0.0290
21·345Y	0.0088
31·245Y	0.0465
32·145Y	0.7921*
41·235Y	0.0302
42·135Y	0.5199*
43·125Y	0.4537*
51·234Y	0.0222
52·134Y	0.3959*
53·124Y	0.3432*
54·123Y	0.8862*

*significant, $P < 0.001$; all others not significant
**coefficient of multiple determination $(r_{Y·12345}^2) = 0.0138$

Y: Normal = 1; Malformed = 2
1: White = 1; Black = 2
2: Maternal age
3: Paternal age
4: Parity
5: Total number of sibs in each sibship

straightforward. For example, the mean maternal age is significantly lower (t_{912} = 2.4518; P < 0.02) in the isolated group, while the mean paternal ages of the 2 groups are nearly identical. Furthermore, the observed maternal and paternal mean ages are lower than the mean age for mutants as estimated by the method of Penrose (1955). Finally, in a multiple regression analysis with "normal" or isolated malformed as the dependent variable and race, maternal age, paternal age, parity, and the total number of sibs in each sibship as the independent variables (Table 7-14) neither maternal age nor paternal age was significantly correlated with being malformed. As expected, though, maternal age, paternal age, parity and total sibs were highly correlated with one another. None of these, however, was correlated with race. These results, then, betray no indication that new mutations are a significant factor in the etiology of sporadic cases.

8. Environmental Variables

Using an analysis of the distribution of congenital malformations, other than the ones being studied, in the sibs of isolated cases and non-malformed, one can attempt to deduce whether there is a teratogenic milieu in the families of sporadic cases responsible for multiple types of malformations, including the malformations under study. A positive answer to this question would suggest that the condition(s) surrounding the teratogenesis were generally extant rather than provisionally unique or private to a given set of pregnancies.

Table 8-1 presents an analysis of the distribution of other congenital malformations in the sibs of isolated cases, familial cases, and non-malformed. As one can see the frequency of malformations was higher in sibs of non-malformed than in sibs of either of the other two groups. Although the frequency is more than 2½ times greater in isolated cases than in familial cases this difference was not significant at the 5% level. This failure to achieve significance may be a reflection of the small sample size, as well as the unavoidable inclusion of nonsporadic cases in the isolated sample. Using an arc sine transformation of the observed frequencies (Sokal and Rohlf, 1969, p. 609) one finds that if one wishes to be 99% certain of detecting a true difference of 0.014 between the two frequencies at the 5% level of significance, about 2682 persons would be needed for each group, familial sibs and isolated sibs. The actual numbers fall far short of this requirement. Nevertheless, comparisons between all three groups did not show significant differences and for this reason alone it is incumbent upon the investigator to search for 1st trimester environmental variables that may be unique to at least the sporadic portion of the isolated group.

TABLE 8-1. Distribution of Other Congenital Malformations in Sibs

Sibs of:	Number Malformed	Number not Malformed	Frequency*
Isolated probands	26	1109	0.02291
Familial probands	1	114	0.00870
Non-malformed	28	906	0.02998

*All comparisons were not significantly different.

THE HEMORRHAGE HYPOTHESIS

As an explanation of human 1st and 2nd branchial arch malformations, Poswillo (1973), using animal models, suggested that the causal mechanism is one of embryonic hematoma formation, the hemorrhage arising from the anastomosis which precedes the formation of the stapedial arterial stem. The anomalies observed ranged from simple reduction of the pinna with or without preauricular tags to complete absence of the external ear with total bony atresia. One of the purposes of this study was to test this hypothesis in humans, particularly those for which no clear genetic etiology could be established. The maternal variables known to cause fetal hemorrhage in animals, and thus studied, were hypertension, pressor agents, salicylates, anticoagulants, and various causes of hypoxia (cigarette smoking, anemia, and chronic lung disease). Since "hemifacial microsomia" was found to be part of the severity spectrum in the animal models, the 2 cases described in Table 6-2 were included in the analysis of this hypothesis for completeness.

The results of this analysis of individual factors are presented in Tables 8-2 through 8-7. Each table contains the observed data in the isolated and non-malformed groups, their respective frequency distributions and the relative risks, which, as defined in Chapter 5, is an indirect estimate of the ratio of the incidence of disease in the exposed group to the incidence of disease in the nonexposed group. Each relative risk ratio is accompanied by a 95% confidence interval.

The frequency of hypertension (Table 8-2), defined as 140+/90+, was not significantly different between the two groups ($\chi^2 = 0.12$; $P > 0.5$). In fact, the frequency was greater in the non-malformed group. Similar results were observed for exposure to pressor agents (Table 8-3) and various degrees of cigarette smoking (Table 8-7). Interestingly, the relative risk of being malformed *decreased* with increasing numbers of cigarettes smoked per day. The relative risks with exposure to salicylates (Table 8-4) and the presence of nutritional anemia (Table 8-5) were

TABLE 8-2. Hypertension and Isolated Cases

	Isolated Probands	Non-malformed*
First trimester hypertension	53	44
No hypertension recorded	472	355
Frequency (%)**	10.09	11.03
Relative risk (RR)	0.91	
95% Confidence limits of RR	0.59 ——————— 1.38	

*1 case no such data recorded
**$\chi_1^2 = 0.12$; $P > 0.5$

TABLE 8-3. Pressor Agents and Isolated Cases

	Isolated Probands	Non-malformed*
First trimester exposure	13	11
No exposure recorded	512	388
Frequency (%)**	2.48	2.75
Relative risk (RR)	0.90	
95% Confidence limits of RR	0.40 ——————— 1.97	

*1 case no such data recorded
**$\chi_1^2 = 0.0032; P > 0.9$

TABLE 8-4. Salicylates and Isolated Cases

	Isolated Probands	Non-malformed
First trimester exposure	158	112
No exposure recorded	367	288
Frequency (%)*	30.09	28.00
Relative risk (RR)	1.11	
95% Confidence limits of RR	0.83 ——————— 1.47	

*$\chi_1^2 = 0.37; P > 0.5$

TABLE 8-5. Nutritional Anemia and Isolated Cases

	Isolated Probands	Non-malformed
First trimester anemia	169	108
No anemia recorded	356	292
Frequency (%)*	32.19	27.00
Relative risk (RR)	1.28	
95% Confidence limits of RR	0.94 ——————— 1.74	

*$\chi_1^2 = 2.67; P > 0.1$

also not statistically significant. The relative risk of being malformed when the mother had chronic lung disease was nearly twice as great in the isolated group as compared to the non-malformed group (Table 8-6). Although this was not significant at the 5% level ($\chi^2 = 1.95$) this may again be a reflection of the sample size. Using the arc sine transformation method presented above, one can determine that in order to be 99% certain of detecting a true difference of .018 between the two frequencies at the 5% level of significance about 3088 persons would be needed for each group, isolated probands and non-malformed.

TABLE 8-6. Chronic Lung Disease* and Isolated Cases

	Isolated Probands	Non-malformed
Present	20	8
Absent	505	392
Frequency (%)**	3.81	2.00
Relative risk (RR)	1.94	
95% Confidence limits of RR	0.83 —————— 4.21	

*Asthma, chronic bronchitis, etc
**$\chi_1^2 = 1.95; P > 0.1$

TABLE 8-7. First Trimester Cigarette Smoking and Isolated Cases

Daily Number Cigarettes Smoked	Isolated Probands	Non-malformed	2X2* χ_1^2	Relative Risk (RR)**	95% Confidence Limits for RR
0	318	206	—	1.00	—
1-4	52	47	1.97	0.72	0.47 - 1.10
5-14	87	63	0.25	0.89	0.62 - 1.29
15-24	57	67	8.32 **	0.55	0.37 - 0.82
25+	11	15	2.76	0.48	0.22 - 1.05

*The relative risk in the absence of cigarette smoking is taken to be 1.00 and all other degrees of cigarette smoking were compared to the 0 group data in χ^2 tests of significance and relative risk calculations.
**$P < 0.005$

These data were further analyzed using combinations of pharmacologic and physiologic risk factors (Table 8-8). Although none of the estimated relative risks were significant for any combination of parameters, the relative risk did increase with the presence of salicylates + pressor agents in combination with hypertension and/or hypoxia. Again the number of pregnancies with such combinations was quite small and much larger groups would be needed to determine if this trend could achieve significance.

Finally, subsequent analyses of these risk factors by race again failed to demonstrate any statistically significant association with the malformations under study, the individual cell sizes becoming very much smaller.

BIRTH ORDER

In a multiple regression analysis (Table 7-14) with "normal" or isolated malformed as the dependent variable and race, maternal age, paternal age, parity and the total number of sibs in each sibship as the independent variables neither parity, maternal age, paternal age, nor total sibs was significantly correlated with being malformed. As expected, though, the independent variables were highly correlated with each other. Parity was not correlated with race; nor were the other independent variables.

TABLE 8-8. Estimated Relative Risks for Variable Combinations as Determined by Isolated Case – Non-malformed Comparisons

Number of Pharmacologic Parameters[a]	Number of Physiologic Parameters[b]		
	0	1	2
0	1.00[c]	0.75	0.94
1	1.00	0.97	0.68
2	0.23	1.35	1.35

[a] salicylates and/or pressor agents

[b] hypertension and/or hypoxia (cigarette smoking, anemia and/or chronic lung disease)

[c] the relative risk in the absence of any parameter is taken to be 1.00 and all parameter combinations were compared to the 0,0 data in tests of significance and relative risk calculations.

SOCIOECONOMIC STATUS

The socioeconomic status in the NCPP population was evaluated by Myrianthopoulos and French (1968) using a technique developed by the U.S. Bureau of the Census. This combines scores for education, occupation and family income to derive a composite numerical profile termed the socioeconomic index (SEI). The index ranges from a low of 0 to a high of 99. These SEI scores represent the socioeconomic status of the child's family at the time of antepartum registration.

The mean SEI and standard error was calculated separately for blacks and whites. The mean score for black isolated cases (34.36 ± 0.85) was significantly lower (t_{584} = 3.5326, P < 0.001) than the mean score for black non-malformed (39.82 ± 1.32). However the mean score for white isolated cases (54.73 ± 2.45) was *not* significantly different (t_{263} = 0.5394, P > 0.5) than the mean score for white non-malformed (56.31 ± 1.66). Interestingly, the socioeconomic index of black familial cases (40.93 ± 2.88) was close to that of black non-malformed. The difference between black familial cases and black isolated cases was close to the 5% level of significance (t_{421} =1.94, P < 0.06). The number of white familial cases was too few (6) to make such a comparison.

The finding of a lower socioeconomic status in a group of affected persons as opposed to nonaffected suggests, in the case of congenital malformations of unknown etiology, the importance of environmental factors, particularly those that are related to nutrition and chronic infectious and noninfectious diseases. Many such variables will be looked at in the remainder of this chapter. It should be pointed out that the number of affected exposed in utero to any given teratogen listed in Tables 8-9 to 8-15 is generally quite small. Since it is well recognized that large sample sizes are needed to detect a teratogenic effect, we sought to maximize the data by combining the races. Also, since the environmental influence is thought to be large vis-a-vis the etiology of the trait (ie most of the isolated cases are sporadic) and the number of black cases is 4 times greater than white cases, any effect that was unique to blacks would tend to inflate the relative risk and would be detected in a subsequent analysis of this factor by race. Although the possibility exists that nonsignificant factors in the combined data may mask a factor unique to white cases, such factors are not likely to achieve statistical significance in any case because of the low frequency of teratogen exposure and the relatively low frequency of the trait in this racial group. This problem is illustrated by the infectious diseases which show that in one case a factor significant in the overall isolated group on subsequent analysis by race achieved significance in blacks only and in another case a factor significant in the total group failed to achieve significance in either racial group alone.

CHRONIC DISEASES DURING PREGNANCY

Table 8-9 lists a variety of chronic diseases found in the mothers of isolated probands and non-malformed during their pregnancy. With the exception of pyelonephritis the relative risk was less than 1 for all diseases studied. Although the estimated relative risk was nearly 2 times greater for those infants whose mothers had pyelonephritis this risk was not statistically significant.

INFECTIOUS DISEASES DURING THE FIRST TRIMESTER

Table 8-10 lists a number of infectious diseases recorded in the mothers of isolated cases and non-malformed during the 1st trimester of pregnancy. Overall there was a significantly increased risk to children whose mothers had either a nonspecific KUB (kidney, ureter, bladder) infection or vaginitis. Analyzed by race, the risk to children whose mothers had a nonspecific KUB infection was only significant for blacks (Table 8-11). Again analyzed separately by race, the risk to children whose mothers had vaginitis during the 1st trimester was *not* statistically significant for either whites or blacks, although the estimated relative risk was nearly 1½ times higher in blacks than in whites (Table 8-12).

TABLE 8-9. Chronic Diseases During Pregnancy

Disease	Isolated Probands (Total = 525)	Non-malformed (Total = 400)	Relative Risk**	95% Confidence Limits
Diabetes mellitus[a]	7(0.0133)*	8(0.0200)	0.66	0.25 - 1.80
Hyperthyroidism	4(0.0076)	4(0.0100)	0.76	0.20 - 2.83
Hypothyroidism	4(0.0076)	8(0.0200)	0.38	0.13 - 1.26
"Epilepsy"[b]	1(0.0019)	1(0.0025)	0.76	0.08 - 7.35
Organic heart disease[c]	10(0.0190)	10(0.0250)	0.76	0.32 - 1.80
Phlebitis	1(0.0019)	2(0.0050)	0.38	0.06 - 3.47
GI disorders[d]	5(0.0095)	8(0.0200)	0.47	0.17 - 1.44
Glomerulonephritis	1(0.0019)	0(0.0000)	undefined	—
Pyelonephritis	5(0.0095)	2(0.0050)	1.91	0.38 - 7.55
Sickle cell anemia	1(0.0019)	1(0.0025)	0.76	0.08 - 7.35

*frequency of the disorder in each study group in parentheses
**no significant differences between study groups

[a] nongestational diabetes mellitus only

[b] noneclamptic convulsive disorders

[c] rheumatic heart disease, congenital heart disease and hypertensive heart disease

[d] peptic ulcer, appendicitis, cholicystitis and cholelithiasis

102 / RESULTS

TABLE 8-10. Infectious Diseases During First Trimester of Pregnancy

Disease	Isolated Proband (Total = 525)	Non-malformed (Total = 400)	Relative Risk	95% Confidence Limits
Influenza	20(0.0381)*	21(0.0525)	0.71	0.38 - 1.33
URI (nonspecific)	135(0.2571)	128(0.3200)	0.74**	0.55 - 0.98
Intestinal parasites	1(0.0019)	2(0.0050)	0.38	0.06 - 3.47
KUB (nonspecific)	113(0.2152)	54(0.1350)	1.76***	1.23 - 2.49
Syphilis	13(0.0248)	12(0.0300)	0.82	0.37 - 5.97
Gonorrhea	3(0.0057)	0(0.0000)	undefined	—
Vaginitis[a]	137(0.2609)	82(0.2050)	1.37**	1.00 - 1.86

*frequency of the disorder in each study group in parentheses
**$P < 0.05$
***$P < 0.005$

[a] monilial, trichomonal, and nonspecific

TABLE 8-11. Nonspecific KUB Infection: Relative Risk by Race

	Isolated Probands	Non-malformed	χ^2_1	Relative Risk	95% Confidence Limits
Black			4.95*	1.68	1.08 - 2.59
KUB infection	102	32			
No KUB infection	303	160			
White			0.005	1.08	0.45 - 2.67
KUB infection	8	14			
No KUB infection	87	164			

*$P < 0.05$

TABLE 8-12. Vaginitis: Relative Risk by Race

	Isolated Probands	Non-malformed	χ^2_1	Relative Risk	95% Confidence Limits
Black			2.24	1.38	0.92 - 2.05
Vaginitis	118	44			
No vaginitis	287	148			
White			0.002	0.96	0.53 - 1.98
Vaginitis	16	31			
No vaginitis	79	147			

MATERNAL VACCINATIONS DURING THE FIRST TRIMESTER

Table 8-13 lists a variety of vaccines administered to mothers during the 1st trimester of their pregnancy. There were no significantly increased relative risks found for any of these vaccines.

OTHER COMPLICATIONS OF PREGNANCY

A number of other pregnancy complications were studied in the mothers of isolated probands and non-malformed and these are listed in Table 8-14. None of these was found to be of significance.

DRUG USE DURING THE FIRST TRIMESTER

Table 8-15 lists a series of specific drugs and classes of drugs that were used by

TABLE 8-13. Maternal Vaccinations During First Trimester of Pregnancy

Vaccine	Isolated Probands (Total = 525)	Non-malformed (Total = 400)	Relative Risk**	95% Confidence Limits
Polio (Sabin)	28(0.0533)*	27(0.0675)	0.78	0.45 - 1.34
Polio (Salk)	42(0.0800)	46(0.1150)	0.67	0.43 - 1.04
Influenza	7(0.0133)	6(0.0150)	0.89	0.31 - 2.53
Tetanus	4(0.0076)	3(0.0075)	1.02	0.24 - 3.99
Diphtheria	1(0.0019)	1(0.0025)	0.76	0.08 - 7.35
Smallpox	1(0.0019)	0(0.0000)	undefined	—
Measles (live)	1(0.0019)	0(0.0000)	undefined	—
Rabies	1(0.0019)	0(0.0000)	undefined	—

*frequency of the disorder in each study group in parentheses
**no significant differences between study groups

TABLE 8-14. Other Complications of Pregnancy

Disorder	Isolated Probands (Total = 525)	Non-malformed (Total = 400)	Relative Risk**	95% Confidence Limits
Hyperemesis gravidarum	2(0.0038)*	3(0.0075)	0.51	0.11 - 2.76
Vaginal bleeding (1st trimester)	80(0.1524)	52(0.1300)	1.20	0.88 - 1.63
Polyhydramnios	3(0.0057)	7(0.0175)	0.32	0.10 - 1.26
Placenta previa	2(0.0038)	3(0.0075)	0.51	0.11 - 2.76
Abruptio placentae	1(0.0019)	3(0.0075)	0.25	0.05 - 2.21
ABO incompatibility[a]	91(0.1904)	68(0.1954)	0.97	0.68 - 1.37
Rh incompatibility[b]	33(0.0690)	20(0.0580)	1.21	0.68 - 2.11

*frequency of the disorder in each study group in parentheses
**no significant differences between study groups

[a] ABO incompatibility data available for 478 isolated probands and 348 non-malformed — frequencies based on these totals

[b] Rh incompatibility data available for 478 isolated probands and 345 non-malformed — frequencies based on these totals

TABLE 8-15. Drug Use During the First Trimester of Pregnancy

Drug	Isolated Proband (Total = 525)	Non-malformed (Total = 400)	Relative Risk**	95% Confidence Limits
Diuretics	2(0.0038)*	6(0.0150)	0.25	0.07 - 1.25
Antihistamines	18(0.0343)	19(0.0475)	0.71	0.37 - 1.37
Barbiturates	18(0.0343)	11(0.0275)	1.26	0.58 - 2.61
Tranquillizers	15(0.0286)	13(0.0325)	0.88	0.41 - 1.83
Penicillin	48(0.0914)	25(0.0625)	1.51	0.91 - 2.46
Tetracycline	4(0.0076)	2(0.0050)	1.53	0.29 - 6.49
Streptomycin	1(0.0019)	1(0.0025)	0.76	0.08 - 7.35
Chloramphenicol	2(0.0038)	1(0.0025)	1.53	0.17 - 9.67
Sulfonamides	2(0.0038)	1(0.0025)	1.53	0.17 - 9.67
Antifungal agents	1(0.0019)	3(0.0075)	0.25	0.05 - 2.21
Insulin	4(0.0076)	5(0.0125)	0.61	0.18 - 2.17
Thyroxin	4(0.0076)	7(0.0175)	0.43	0.14 - 1.47
Estrogen	6(0.0114)	9(0.0225)	0.50	0.19 - 1.41
Progesterone	11(0.0209)	10(0.0250)	0.83	0.36 - 1.94

*frequency of the disorder in each study group in parentheses
**no significant differences between study groups

mothers of isolated cases and non-malformed. Although none of these drugs presented a statistically significant risk to the unborn fetus, it is still interesting to note that the estimated relative risks were, with the exception of streptomycin, uniformly 1½ times greater for those exposed in utero to antibacterials. Because of the relatively larger sample sizes and narrower 95% confidence interval, penicillin may be of particular importance.

GENE-ENVIRONMENT INTERACTION: TWINS

There are 188 monozygotic twin pairs in the NCPP population for whom information about the presence or absence of malformations is available. Of these, 4 had 1 twin with isolated nonsyndromic external ear malformations (2 with unilateral preauricular sinuses and 2 with unilateral preauricular tags). This is an incidence of 2.13%, not significantly different ($\chi_1^2 = 1.19$, $P > 0.1$) from the singleton population incidence of 1.05%. The laterality was evenly divided between right and left, and all 4 were females. Two pairs were black, 1 white, and 1 Puerto Rican. The proband concordance rate was 0%.

There are 309 dizygotic twin pairs in the NCPP population for whom information about the presence or absence of malformations is available. Of these, 8 had at least 1 twin with isolated nonsyndromic external ear malformations (2 twins with preauricular tags and 7 with preauricular sinuses). This is an incidence of 2.59%, a frequency not significantly different from the expected frequency of 2.09% as calculated from a two-element binomial expansion and the frequency in singletons. There were 3 DZ twins with bilateral ear malformations, and 6 with unilateral malformations, 3 left and 3 right. The male/female ratio was 5 to 4. Seven of the affected DZ twin pairs were black and 1 white. These 8 twin pairs represented 1 concordant pair and 7 discordant pairs, a proband concordance rate of 22%. It is of note that 1 member of the concordant pair had bilateral malformations and the other had a unilateral left malformation. This concordant pair was black and of unlike sex.

These data tend to support the hypothesis that the relative contribution of genetic factors to the etiology of isolated nonsyndromic external ear malformations is not large.

9. Natural History

Little is known about the natural history of those children who have nonsyndromic isolated or familial external ear and/or branchial cleft malformations. There are some indications that congenital hearing loss is likely to be an important factor (Harada and Ishii, 1972; Jaffe, 1976). Furthermore, Hanson et al (1976) pointed out that prenatal growth deficiency is the most consistent single feature of major known teratogens yet recognized in man, being expressed as abnormal skeletal and psychomotor development. This factor may be of particular importance with regard to the sporadic cases in this study. In order to evaluate all these possibilities several variables were investigated including prenatal growth deficiency (low birthweight), intelligence (IQ), hearing loss, and abnormal speech production in the absence of deafness, mental retardation, and speech mechanism anomalies.

BIRTHWEIGHT AND ISOLATED EXTERNAL EAR MALFORMATIONS

In order to examine the possible effects of a less than optimum (teratogenic) in utero environment on the somatic and physiologic development of infants with isolated cases of external ear and/or branchial cleft malformations a number of factors were considered, namely birthweight, Apgar score, and gestational age. Obviously some of these variables are likely to be correlated with each other and perhaps with race. Thus it was decided that the most appropriate analysis was a multiple regression analysis with non-malformed or malformed as the dependent variable, and race, Apgar score, birthweight, and gestational age as the independent variables. The results are presented in Table 9-1. As we can see, birthweight, when the other independent variables were held constant, was not significantly correlated with malformation; similarly, neither were gestational age nor Apgar score. Race, as expected, was associated with malformation. With regard to race it is interesting to note here that a black infant, non-malformed or malformed, was more likely to have a lower birthweight and a lower gestational age (both of which are highly correlated) but a higher Apgar score.

These data betray no indication that prenatal growth deficiency expressed as low birthweight is a significant factor in children with isolated external ear and/or branchial cleft malformation.

TABLE 9-1. Gestational Age, Birthweight, and Apgar Score: Regression Analysis

PARTIAL CORRELATIONS	PARTIAL COEFFICIENTS**
1Y·234	0.3071*
2Y·134	0.0552
3Y·124	-0.0517
4Y·123	-0.0231
21·34Y	0.1450*
31·24Y	-0.1051*
32·14Y	0.0386
41·23Y	-0.0926*
42·13Y	0.0681
43·12Y	0.4063*

*significant, $P < 0.05$; all others not significant
**coefficient of multiple determination ($r^2_{y \cdot 1234}$) = 0.0950

Y: Non-malformed = 1; Malformed = 2
1: White = 1; Black = 2
2: Apgar score
3: Birthweight (grams)
4: Gestational age (weeks)

INTELLIGENCE (IQ)

IQ was measured at age 4 years with the abbreviated version of the Stanford-Binet Intelligence Scale (Form L-M) and at age 7 years with the Wechsler Intelligence Scale for Children (WISC). It has been shown previously that the best predictors of 4 year IQ in the NCPP population, blacks and whites, are socioeconomic status and the Bayley motor and mental scores at 8 months of age (Broman et al, 1975). Thus, since it is known that the NCPP population blacks have considerably lower socioeconomic index scores than whites (see Chapter 8, and Myrianthopoulos and French, 1968), blacks and whites are considered separately.

As shown in Table 9-2, the frequency of mental retardation (IQ ≤ 69) in white isolated cases was not significantly different from that in the white non-malformed population. The same was true of blacks. Since the number of familial cases was small further stratification into black/white racial groups was not possible. Nevertheless, the frequency of mental retardation in the total of black and white familial cases was not significantly different from that in the combined black and white non-malformed population (Table 9-3).

Viewing IQ overall at age 7 years (Table 9-4) it can be seen that the mean IQ of white isolated cases was not significantly different from the white non-malformed group. The same was true for blacks. The mean IQ for black familial cases (91.04 ±

TABLE 9-2. Mental Retardation and Isolated External Ear Malformations

		ISOLATED CASES		NON-MALFORMED
White	Mental retardation	3		3
	IQ > 69	92		175
	2 × 2 χ^2		0.13	
Black	Mental retardation	16		13
	IQ > 69	389		179
	2 × 2 χ^2		1.67	
Combined	Mental retardation	19		16
	IQ > 69	481		354
	2 × 2 χ^2		0.05	

All χ^2 values not significant

TABLE 9-3. Mental Retardation and Familial External Ear Malformations

	FAMILIAL CASES		NON-MALFORMED
Mental retardation	1		16
IQ > 69	34		354
2 × 2 χ^2		0.001	

TABLE 9-4. 7 Year IQ and Isolated External Ear Malformations

| | MEAN ± SE | | | |
RACE	ISOLATED CASES	NON-MALFORMED	DF	t VALUE
White	100.01 ± 1.87	102.24 ± 1.20	227	1.02
Black	90.97 ± 1.86	89.42 ± 0.94	533	0.58

DF = degrees of freedom

2.54) was also not significantly different (t_{393} = 0.59) from the black non-malformed group and the same was true of whites (mean for cases = 108.75 ± 13.58; t_{159} = 0.83), although the number of white familial cases (4) with 7 year IQ scores was very small.

These data suggest that the etiologic agents associated with familial and isolated external ear and/or branchial cleft malformations have no detectable effect on the mental developmental of affected infants, black or white.

HEARING

Audiologic screening by various methods was performed on the NCPP study children on numerous occasions. Detailed audiologic testing was carried out at ages 3 and 8, including pure-tone audiometry. A loss of greater than 15 db was considered abnormal. Among the isolated cases, adequate 8-year pure-tone audiometry was completed for 77 of 95 whites and 369 of 405 blacks. Among the non-malformed group, the same data were available for 172 of 178 whites and 186 of 192 blacks. For familial cases 28 of 33 were so tested. Comparisons between affected and non-malformed groups are given in Table 9-5. The frequency of abnormal hearing loss of all kinds was significantly greater ($P < 0.05$) in isolated white cases than in white non-malformed. This was not the case for blacks although the frequency in the black cases (10%) was twice that found in the black non-malformed. Looking at the combined (ie black and white) familial cases (Table 9-6) again we can see that the frequency of abnormal hearing loss is almost identical with that found in the combined white/black non-malformed group ($\chi^2 = 0.09$).

In order to characterize the laterality and nature of the hearing loss in the malformed cases, as well as the ipsilaterality or contralaterality to the malformed ear, an attempt was made to list the hearing loss by side in one of three broad categories, conductive, sensorineural and mixed. The category of hearing loss was either specifically stated in the patient's chart or determined by us according to the criteria set forth in Newby (1964). In short, a patient with a conductive loss presents an audiogram showing losses by air conduction (pathology of the outer and/or middle ear) but normal hearing by bone conduction. Sensorineural hearing loss (pathology of the inner ear) is characterized usually, but not always, by greater losses at the higher frequencies. In this type of loss the bone-conduction thresholds are approximately the same as the air-conduction thresholds. A mixed hearing loss shows some loss by bone conduction. It may also present as a conductive loss in the lower frequencies and sensorineural loss in the higher frequencies. Those cases in which only air-conduction audiometry was done were classified as "type unknown."

The two familial cases with hearing loss both had bilateral conductive impairment. One case had bilateral preauricular sinuses and the other bilateral anomalies of the helix and antihelix.

Of the 52 isolated cases with hearing loss, 11 were "type unknown." Of the remainder, 29 (71%) had conductive hearing loss, 8 (19%) sensorineural hearing loss, and 4 (10%) mixed hearing loss. Viewed another way, a conductive component was present in 81% of the cases with hearing loss and a sensorineural component in 29%. There were 20 cases (38%) in which there was a hearing loss contralateral to the ear with the malformation, 8 of these 20 (40%) having no hearing loss on the ipsilateral side. All

TABLE 9-5. Hearing Loss and Isolated External Ear Malformations

		ISOLATED CASES	NON-MALFORMED
White	Hearing loss	14	14
	Normal	63	158
	$2 \times 2\ \chi^2$	4.42*	
Black	Hearing loss	38	10
	Normal	331	176
	$2 \times 2\ \chi^2$	3.19	
Combined	Hearing loss	52	24
	Normal	394	334
	$2 \times 2\ \chi^2$	5.13*	

*significant, $P < 0.05$

TABLE 9-6. Hearing Loss and Familial External Ear Malformations

	FAMILIAL CASES	NON-MALFORMED
Hearing loss	2	24
Normal	26	334
$2 \times 2\ \chi^2$	0.09	

these data are presented in Table 9-7. There are 4 points of great interest here: 1) the surprising number of unilateral external ear malformations with unilateral (mostly ipsilateral) sensorineural hearing loss; 2) all 4 cases of mixed hearing loss are bilateral regardless of the unilaterality of the external ear malformations; 3) only 1 of the 2 cases of "hemifacial microsomia" had a hearing loss and that was bilateral sensorineural; 4) of the 11 cases of nonsyndromic branchial cleft sinuses, there were no instances of a hearing loss. These data would strongly suggest considerable dysmorphic asymmetry of the external, middle and inner ear structures for each individual patient as well as great phenotypic variability among those patients who demonstrated a hearing loss.

TABLE 9-7. Isolated Cases, Hearing Loss, and Relative Laterality

WHITES

EXTERNAL EAR MALFORMATIONS	HEARING LOSS
L-PAS	L-S
B-PAS	B-C
R-PAS	B-TU
R-PAT	B-S
R-PAT	B-C
L-PAT, R-DP	R-C
R-PAT, R-DP	R-S
R-DP	B-TU
B-DP	L-C
R-MIC	R-TU
R-MIC	R-C
R-MIC	R-C
B-DP	B-C
HM	B-S

BLACKS

EXTERNAL EAR MALFORMATIONS	HEARING LOSS
B-PAS	B-TU
L-PAS	L-S
L-PAS	B-C
B-PAS	B-TU
R-PAS	L-TU
L-PAS	L-C
R-PAS	R-C
B-PAS	B-C
B-DP, L-PAS	L-C
L-PAS	B-S
R-PAS	R-S
B-PAS	L-C

B-PAS	R-C
B-PAS	B-TU
R-PAS	L-TU
L-PAS	B-M
R-PAS	B-C
B-PAS	L-C
R-PAS	L-C
R-PAS	R-C
B-PAS	B-M
R-PAS	L-C
L-PAS	B-C
L-PAS	R-C
R-PAS	L-C
R-PAS	L-C
R-PAS	B-M
L-PAS	L-C
R-MIC	R-C
B-MIC	B-C
R-MIC	R-C
L-PAT	L-C
B-PAT	R-TU
L-PAT, R-PAS	B-TU
L-PAT	L-TU
R-PAT	L-S
R-PAS	B-M
L-PAS	L-C

L = left; R = right; B = bilateral; PAS = preauricular sinus; PAT = preauricular tag; MIC = microtia; DP = other pinna malformations; C = conductive hearing loss; S = sensorineural hearing loss; M = mixed hearing loss; TU = unknown type of hearing loss (bone conduction studies not done).

SPEECH PRODUCTION

Evaluation of the speech mechanism and speech production was performed in detail at ages 3 and 8 years. Among the isolated cases sufficient data were available for 77 of 95 whites and 384 of 405 blacks. Among non-malformed the same studies were completed for 172 of 178 whites and 189 of 192 blacks. For familial cases 32 of 33 were so tested. Comparisons between affected and non-malformed groups are given in Table 9-8. It is important to remember that the speech anomalies considered here are only those of speech production in the absence of hearing loss, mental retardation, and speech mechanism pathology. The frequency of such speech production anomalies (disarticulation) in white isolated cases was significantly greater ($P < 0.05$) than that in the white non-malformed group. This was very much different in the blacks where the frequency for isolated cases was not significantly different from the non-malformed ($P > 0.1$). Looking at the combined familial cases (Table 9-9) we can see that the frequencies of abnormal speech articulation were not significantly different than those found in the combined white/black non-malformed group ($\chi_1^2 = 0.99, P > 0.1$).

TABLE 9-8. Speech Articulation and Isolated External Ear Malformations

		ISOLATED CASES		NON-MALFORMED
White	Abnormal	11		10
	Normal	66		162
	$2 \times 2 \chi^2$		3.91*	
Black	Abnormal	45		18
	Normal	339		171
	$2 \times 2 \chi^2$		0.42	
Combined	Abnormal	56		28
	Normal	405		333
	$2 \times 2 \chi^2$		3.79**	

*signifigant, $P < 0.05$
**$p \approx 0.05$

TABLE 9-9. Speech Articulation and Familial External Ear Malformations

	FAMILIAL CASES		NON-MALFORMED
Abnormal	4		28
Normal	22		333
$2 \times 2 \chi^2$		0.99	

PART IV
DISCUSSION AND SUMMARY

10. Discussion

It is apparent that malformations of the external ear (including branchial cleft sinuses) are common, the birth incidence being about 1%. After reviewing the literature we concluded that the reported within-family, as well as "within-person," variability of these malformations is quite considerable whether we investigate single monogenic traits or syndromes. This variability was also seen in the experimental animal models (Poswillo, 1973). Thus, prior to the present investigation there was some reason to believe that a single etiologic factor may be associated with a variety of ear malformations even in one individual. This hypothesis has been given considerable support by the analysis of the NCPP data (Tables 6-4 and 6-5). From these data it would appear that multiple external ear and/or branchial cleft malformations in a single individual are more likely associated with "multiple hits" by a single etiology and that any given malformation of the type studied here is not necessarily etiologically distinct from any other of this type. This, of course, in no way denies etiologic heterogeneity for the group as a whole. Finally, the embryologic and teratologic evidence presented in Chapter 1 would seem to support the idea that external ear and branchial cleft malformations are associated with a breakdown in neural crest integrity, more often than not the result of aberrant crest-cell migration and/or pre- or postdifferentiation viability. If the primary etiology is genetic, the phenotypic variability will be a function of the so-called "genetic background" and environmental milieu; if the primary etiology is environmental, the phenotypic variability will depend upon the capacity of the involved tissues to repair and redifferentiate before the processes of programmed differentiation shut off toward the end of embryogenesis (Poswillo, 1973), and this capacity will also be a function of the genetic background and remaining environmental milieu.

RACIAL VARIABILITY

The birth incidence of external ear and/or branchial cleft malformations was more than 4 times greater in blacks than in whites, and this was highly significant

118 / DISCUSSION AND SUMMARY

(Table 6-11). This was true for both familial and isolated cases and this racial variation in frequency was independent of the institutional variation (Table 6-14). Although blacks were more likely to have preauricular sinuses than whites, they generally had the same or greater frequencies of the other phenotypes as well (Table 6-12). This racial phenotypic variability may be a function of the relative frequencies of varying etiologies. Support for this can be found in the fact that 1) the heritability estimate in whites was 185 times higher than in blacks, and 2) the mean socioeconomic index score for black isolated cases was significantly lower than the mean score for black non-malformed, while this was not so for whites. Interestingly the only specific environmental variable that was found to be statistically significant in this study, KUB infections, was significant for blacks only. In addition, the frequency of hearing and speech articulation anomalies was only significant in the white isolated cases, further hinting at possible differences in the relative frequencies of as yet unknown etiologies.

GENETIC CONSIDERATIONS

As presented in Tables 7-1, 7-2 and 7-3 the multifactorial/threshold inheritance analysis for both blacks and whites demonstrated: 1) the observed incidence in 1° relatives of probands does not conform with the predictions of the model; 2) the severity of the proband's malformation and/or the number of affected up to and including the proband has no apparent relationship to the risk of recurrence in future sibs. In addition, the heritability estimates are low in both races, particularly so in blacks. Thus, the classic multifactorial/threshold model which includes polygenic inheritance is an unsatisfactory explanation of these data. This is not surprising since this model has, in the real world of dysmorphology, been more an illusion than a contingency (Kidd and Spence, 1976; Melnick and Shields, 1976; Melnick et al, 1977).

Since the multifactorial/threshold model was not adequate as an etiologic explanation of the NCPP external ear malformation data, it became necessary to search for alternatives. The alternative that came to mind was the possibility that the familial cases were primarily genetic in etiology and the isolated cases were primarily nongenetic in etiology. To support this contention there are a number of parameters which distinguish the familial group of probands from the isolated group. These include: 1) the frequency of bilateral cases is considerably greater in the familial group than the isolated group; 2) in the familial group alone, there is a slight excess of affected females which is complimented by a significant excess of unaffected males; 3) at least in blacks, there is a significantly lower socioeconomic index (SEI) score for isolated cases when compared to the non-malformed group but the SEI score in familial cases is not significantly different from the non-malformed group; 4) there is an increased frequency of single additional malformations of many kinds in the isolated cases alone; 5) the frequency of hearing loss and abnormal speech articulation was significantly elevated in the isolated cases but not the familial cases when compared to the non-malformed group. These dichotomies and the fact that half the families of familial probands demonstrated vertical transmission through 2 and 3 generations (including male-to-male) made it reasonable to regard at least the familial cases as likely monogenic cases. Nevertheless, there exists the very real possibility that some proportion of the isolated cases are in fact the affected children of nonpenetrant gene carrier parents and an estimate of these was sought with the aid of SEGRAN (Morton, 1959).

These NCPP data indicate that there is a substantial number of isolated cases which are in fact chance isolated and not sporadic. It is interesting that this was so for both racial groups. It is also noteworthy that the segregation frequency as estimated from various race-mating type groups (black U X U, black A X U, and white U X U) was consistently about 10-13%. Given these findings and the estimated gene frequencies under alternative sets of assumptions (Tables 7-11 and 7-12), one might reasonably conclude that the etiology of the familial cases is an autosomal gene, common recessive or less common dominant, with very low penetrance. One must admit, however, that since the heritabilities are quite low in both races and the frequency of external ear malformations is the same in black 1° relatives as in the general population, to some this explanation may not be entirely satisfying. Certainly one could make a case for nongenetic etiologies alone. However, there does exist the possibility that environmental induction of external ear anomalies is associated with a monogenic susceptibility to the environment, ie manifestation being dependent upon environmental triggers as well as a single mutant gene (Penrose, 1953). The familial clustering of affected persons, then, could be due to the fact that close relatives are more genetically alike and are more likely to share common environments (dietary habits, hygiene habits, etc). Indeed, this may be an alternative explanation for all cases, both isolated and familial.

GENETIC COUNSELING

Although it would be of great benefit to know more precisely the etiology of all cases of nonsyndromic external ear malformations, one can still reasonably formulate recurrence risks with the somewhat empiric risk data provided by this study.

We are generally confronted with 4 kinds of families: 1) simplex, unaffected parents, negative family history; 2) simplex, one affected parent; 3) multiplex, unaffected parents, negative family history; 4) multiplex, one affected parent. In the *first family type* one may use Tables 7-6 and 7-10 to calculate the probability that an isolated case is sporadic and then multiply the remainder by a segregation frequency of 10% to get the recurrence risk for subsequent sibs. For example, in a two-child black family the risk would be (1-0.819) (10%) or about 2%. In family types 2, 3 and 4 listed above it is reasonable to assume that these cases are genetic and the risk to subsequent sibs will be about 10%.

ENVIRONMENTAL CONSIDERATIONS

Undoubtedly the low level of genetic determination for the trait in the NCPP population as a whole (particularly in blacks) and the significantly lower socioeconomic status of black isolated cases speak for a strong environmental input in the etiology of external ear malformations.

With this in mind a large number of environmental factors were investigated with disappointing but not unexpected results. Factors relating to the "hemorrhage hypothesis" (Poswillo, 1973) were studied, and, with the exception of chronic lung disease, all estimated relative risk ratios were close to unity. In all cases there were no statistically significant risk ratios. With the exception of KUB infections, the same was true for a whole series of other maternal factors studied. It should be noted, however, that the 95% confidence limits were considerably wide for many of these parameters and thus it is not totally possible to rule out a teratogenic effect for at least those in which the risk ratio was well above 1, such as pyelonephritis (Table 8-9), vaginitis (Table 8-10), Rh incompatibility (Table 8-14), a number of antibiotics (Table 8-15), and barbiturates (Table 8-15). Nevertheless, if such an effect is present the data suggest that it is not likely to be a strong one and a much larger sample size would be needed to detect it. Since this is not likely to be available in the near future, animal studies might be profitable for some of the parameters just mentioned.

Concerning the increased risk to children whose mothers have 1st trimester KUB infections, the meaning remains obscure to us. Since this was found only in blacks it may be related to the significantly lowered socioeconomic status. For this reason, as well as chance alone, this finding may be spurious. On the other hand, this finding could be real and possibly related to the effects of hyperthermia (Poswillo et al, 1974).

Finally it should be noted that a failure to clearly identify any environmental risk factors may be due in part to our inability to eliminate the chance isolated (presumed genetic) cases from the total isolated case sample. Nevertheless, until such time as we can identify, positively, such chance isolated cases, we are forced to either accept this epidemiologic pollution or not do the analysis at all.

SYNDROME IDENTIFICATION

What follows is a classification of the major single anomalies, syndromes and statistically significant associations that involve external ear and/or branchial cleft malformations. Syndromes are classified according to guidelines suggested by Cohen (1977):

A. Syndromes of uncertain etiology
   1. Provisionally-unique pattern syndrome
   2. Recurrent pattern syndrome
B. Syndromes of known etiology
   1. Pedigree syndrome
   2. Chromosomal syndrome
   3. Environmentally-induced syndrome

The syndromes that are included in this listing are only those in which we feel that the external ear and/or branchial cleft malformations are so striking as to cause the clinician to consider them first in the differential. This is somewhat subjective and perhaps tautologic but so be it.

The terms used in this classification are defined as follows:
1) *single malformation:* a primary structural defect (tissue or organ) that results from a localized error of morphogenesis (Smith, 1976).
2) *deformation:* an alteration in shape and/or structure of a previously normally formed part (Smith 1976).
3) *provisionally-unique pattern syndrome:* "two or more abnormalities in the same patient such that the clinician does not recognize the overall pattern of defects from his own experience, nor from searching the literature, nor from consultation with the most learned colleagues in the field" (Cohen, 1977).
4) *recurrent pattern syndrome:* "a similar or identical set of abnormalities in two or more unrelated patients" (Cohen, 1977).
5) *pedigree syndrome:* "known genesis established on the basis of pedigree evidence alone; the basic defect itself remains undefined although it is known to represent a monogenic disorder" (Cohen, 1977); does not exclude the possibility that manifestation depends on important environmental triggers.
6) *chromosomal syndrome:* cytogenetically defined.
7) *environmentally-induced syndrome:* defined in terms of the known associated environmental teratogen; does not exclude the possibility of genetic susceptibility to a given environment.
8) *association syndrome:* a weak recurrent pattern syndrome in which usually two malformations are positively correlated statistically (Cohen, 1977). The etiology is obscure.

Cohen (1977) makes 2 very important points about these defined terms. First, the use of these terms in syndrome delineation should never be thought of as static, immutable categories but rather as a dynamic, flexible and continually changing framework in which to view various syndromes. Second, one must be careful not to confuse syndrome delineation with an understanding or lack thereof of the syndrome's pathogenesis even at the higher stages of delineation. To assume otherwise is at best misleading unless supported by additional evidence.

CLASSIFICATION OF EXTERNAL EAR AND/OR BRANCHIAL CLEFT MALFORMATIONS

A. Single malformations
  1. Known etiology* (genetic: ?AD or AR)**
     a) ear pits
     b) ear tags
     c) anotia/microtia
     d) other malformed pinna (lop, cup, protruding, etc)
     e) branchial cleft sinus or fistula
  2. Uncertain etiology*
     a) ear pits
     b) ear tags
     c) anotia/microtia
     d) cryptotia
     e) lobule coloboma or agenesis
     f) other malformed pinna (lop, cup, protruding, etc)
     g) branchial cleft sinus or fistula
B. Deformation
  Oligohydramniotic postural molding (Potter syndrome → large, flattened auricles)
C. Syndromes of known etiology (see Chapters 1-3)
  1. Pedigree syndrome
     a) Mandibulofacial dysostosis (AD)
     b) Konigsmark-Gorlin otomandibular dysostosis (AD)
     c) branchio-oto dysplasia (AD)
     d) microtia-meatal atresia—conductive hearing loss syndrome (AR)
     e) hypertrophic ear lobes—conductive hearing loss (Escher-Hirt) syndrome (AD)
     f) branchio-oto-renal dysplasia (AD)
     g) dysplastic pinna-hypospadias-renal adysplasia syndrome (AD)
     h) dysplastic pinna-polycystic kidney syndrome (AD)
     i) oto-renal-genital syndrome (AR)
     j) auriculo-osteodysplasia syndrome (AD)
     k) Bixler syndrome (AR)
     l) LADD syndrome (AD)
     m) Mengel syndrome (AR)
     n) oto-facio-cervical syndrome (AD)
     o) Townes-Brocks syndrome (AD)

*There is strong evidence that these malformations may not necessarily be etiologically distinct.
**AD = autosomal dominant; AR = autosomal recessive.

2. Chromosomal syndrome
     a) 4p- syndrome
     b) trisomy 11 syndrome
     c) Cat-eye syndrome (probably trisomy 22)
  3. Environmentally-induced
     a) Thalidomide syndrome
     b) Amniotic band syndrome
D. Syndromes of uncertain etiology
  1. Provisionally-unique pattern syndromes
     See Table 6-2; it is our hope that others will recognize these in their own patient populations and elevate them to recurrent pattern syndrome status
  2. Recurrent pattern syndromes
     a) 1st and 2nd branchial arch syndrome
     b) otocephaly syndrome
  3. Association syndromes: external ear malformations and . . .
     a) craniosynostosis
     b) kyphoscoliosis
     c) pectus carinatum
     d) congenital heart disease
     e) inguinal hernia
     f) dysmorphic ureters
     g) minor digital dysmorphia
     h) strawberry/port wine hemangiomas
     i) pigmented nevi
     j) café-au-lait spots
     k) vitiligo

The single malformations of "known" etiology tend to occur bilaterally more often than those of unknown etiology. Of the unilateral cases, "known" or unknown etiology, there is a marked predilection for the right side. Although the reason for this is unclear, it may be related to laterality differences in embryonic blood supply.

Finally, there are a few points to be made about some of the syndromes. First, present evidence suggests that branchio-oto dysplasia and branchio-oto-renal dysplasia are distinct entities (Melnick et al, 1978). The phenotypic expression of the branchial, audiologic and renal anomalies can be quite variable, even within the same family. It is important that both renal and audiologic studies be carried out in all patients with familial branchial arch malformations because of the clinical implications of an unrecognized prelingual hearing loss and the prognostic importance for genetic counseling if renal malformations are found. Second, the parents and sibs of infants with "Potter facies" in the presence of auricular malformation and renal adysplasia should be carefully scrutinized for any evidence of branchial arch malformations, hearing loss, or renal anomalies in order to rule out a heritable ear dysplasia-renal adysplasia syndrome. Third, a newborn who dies in the neonatal period or shortly thereafter with the Potter facies/branchio-oto-renal dysplasia phenotype (Fitch and Srolovitz, 1976; Melnick et al, 1978) should be considered as a possible trisomy 11 (Blair, 1976) until demonstrated otherwise. Fourth, the birth incidence of some of the more common "external ear syndromes" has been estimated from the NCPP population as follows: Potter syndrome (sans true extrarenal malformations) 1/53000; mandibulofacial dysostosis 1/27000; branchio-oto dysplasia 1/53000; 1st and 2nd branchial arch (FSBA) syndrome 1/27000. The last estimate may be too low since many of the unilateral microtias and other external ear malformations listed as single malformations may in fact represent the mildest form of the 1st and 2nd branchial arch syndrome. Conversely, the FSBA syndrome may be the most severe effect of teratogens that also initiate more mild external ear malformations and such nosologic division by severity may be unjustified.

NATURAL HISTORY

In the past, two abnormalities have been frequently associated with external ear malformations: conductive hearing loss associated with middle ear anomalies, and malformation of the urinary tract. As Jaffe (1976) pointed out, however, external ear malformations are far more commonly associated with middle ear anomalies (conductive hearing loss) than with urinary tract anomalies. This clinical observation by Jaffe (1976) has been substantiated by the NCPP data, at least as it relates to dysfunctional anomalies of the urinary tract. The frequency of a conductive component hearing loss among the isolated probands in the NCPP population was about 6%, while the frequency of dysfunctional urinary tract anomalies (dysmorphic ureters) was about 0.4%. This, however, does not minimize the importance of the latter finding.

Regarding the hearing loss there were several surprising findings. First, the frequency of hearing loss in familial, presumed monogenic, cases of external ear malformations was not significantly different from the non-malformed population. The opposite was found in the isolated cases. Second, more than 1/3 of the isolated cases with hearing loss had a loss contralateral to the ear with the malformation, 40% of these having no hearing loss of the ipsilateral side. Third, nearly 1/3 of the isolated cases with hearing loss had a sensorineural component.

These data require some interesting speculations if the hemorrhage hypothesis (Poswillo, 1973) is to be maintained as relevant to the human condition. It was pointed out by Grabb (1965) that in his study of 102 1st and 2nd branchial arch malformation patients none had inner ear involvement. He speculated that the reason for this was that the inner ear is protected from damage induced by teratogens that affect the external and middle ear by the prior existence of the precartilaginous otic capsule. However, it is known that hematoma formation can deform nose cartilage in diphenylhydantoin treated mice (K.S. Brown, personal communication). If the expanding hematoma theory is true, then the NCPP data would also suggest that this protection is often not forthcoming in man. Similarly Naunton and Valvassori (1968) found that 12% of a series of patients with external auditory meatal atresia had inner ear abnormalities. They also found that these anomalies varied in type and were both ipsilateral and contralateral to the meatal atresia. This raises a second point: that is, if the hemorrhage mechanism is operative in man then there is either considerable repair and redifferentiation of the external and/or middle ear structures or the hematomas often expand medially without expanding laterally. Either possibility would explain the unexpectedly large number of NCPP cases with hearing loss contralateral to the external ear malformation. It should be pointed out that although these NCPP data strongly suggest considerable dysmorphic asymmetry of the external, middle and inner ear structures this is not entirely inconsistent with Poswillo's (1973) animal model. Nevertheless, his failure to produce inner ear anomalies remains a mystery.

Perhaps the most interesting findings in the NCPP population with isolated external ear malformations are the significantly increased incidence of skin pigmentation anomalies (nevi, café-au-lait spots and vitiligo), and speech production anomalies (disarticulation) in the absence of hearing loss, mental retardation, and speech mechanism pathology. In light of these findings, along with that of sensorineural hearing loss, it is tempting to speculate that at least some of the isolated cases may represent an earlier, more basic defect in the neuroectoderm prior to or at the time of development of the neural crest.

Neural crest cells that migrate from the area of the primitive rhombencephalon move around the anterolateral margin of the 1st pharyngeal pouch into the presumptive 1st and 2nd branchial arches and provide the major contribution to the development of the external and middle ear structures (Noden, 1975). Ectomesenchymal neural crest cells are also the precursors of glial and Schwann sheath cells as well as pigment cells (LeDouarin, 1975; Noden, 1975). It has recently been shown that the neural crest participates in the formation of a number of receptors, among which is the auditory receptor epithelium (Johnston et al, 1975). In this case the function of the crest cells appears to be concerned with the regulation of inner ear fluid (endolymph) which is essential to maintaining the electrical potential for stimulation of inner ear hair cells. In addition, there are a number of mouse mutants (eg piebald-lethal) which suggest abnormalities of the neural crest before its differentiation, resulting in abnormalities of pigmentation and dysplasias of the acoustic ganglion (Deol, 1968).

The common denominator, then, in the pathogenesis of these anomalies may indeed be intrinsic or environmental abnormalities of premigratory neural crest tissue, particularly in the area of the primitive rhombencephalon but not restricted to it. It is now known that cephalic neural crest cells are pluripotential with respect to their migratory behavior, and that the patterns of their migrations are largely under the control of local environmental influences (Noden, 1975). Perhaps the origin of the pathogenesis of many of the cases of external ear malformations can be found in this local environment.

11. Summary

Using data from the prospective NINCDS Collaborative Perinatal Project (NCPP) (N = 53,257), 558 children, who were found to have nonsyndromic auricular anomalies ranging in severity from preauricular pits and tags to bilateral microtia, were compared to 400 randomly selected non-malformed children.

The frequency of external ear malformations was 1.72% in blacks and 0.42% in whites. Chi-square analysis revealed that various types of ear malformations occurred together more often than by chance and that such combinations were more likely the consequence of multiple hits by single etiologies. Thus any given malformation of the type studied is not necessarily etiologically distinct from any other of this type.

The M/F sex ratio was 1.06 for familial probands, 1.11 for isolated probands, and 1.11 overall. The frequency of bilateral ear malformations was considerably greater in the familial cases than the isolated cases. Regarding unilateral malformation, there was a significant predilection for the right side. The frequency of a single additional malformation in the isolated cases was significantly greater than the malformation frequency in the remaining NCPP population. This was not so for familial cases. Specifically, the anomalies that were significantly associated with isolated cases were craniosynostosis, kyphoscoliosis, pectus carinatum, congenital heart disease, inguinal hernia, dysmorphic ureters, mild digital dysmorphia, strawberry/port wine hemangioma, pigmented nevi, café-au-lait spots, and vitiligo. Among familial cases only lacrimal duct stenosis was significantly elevated.

Pedigree data for the probands were collected prior to birth and again at age 7 years. The frequency of familial cases among all cases was 6% in both blacks and whites. Tests for multifactorial/threshold inheritance gave a poor fit and this hypothesis was ultimately discarded as an explanation of the data. Segregation analysis, by race, of all cases was accomplished by the SEGRAN method (Morton, 1959) which provides maximum likelihood estimates of $\emptyset$ (segregation probability), χ (proportion of sporadic cases), and π (ascertainment probability). *For blacks,* iteration on all Normal X Normal (NXN) matings (N = 413) yielded as best estimates $\emptyset$ = 10%, χ = 80%, and π = 75%. Iteration on all Affected X Normal (AXN) matings (N = 10) yielded as best estimates $\emptyset = 13\%$, $\chi = 0\%$, $\pi = 100\%$. *For whites,* iteration on all N×N matings gave best estimates of $\emptyset = 10\%$, $\chi = 83\%$, and $\pi = 36\%$. Unfortunately there were only 3 A×N matings. A Weinberg Proband Method calculation estimated $\emptyset = 14\%$, consistent with the results in blacks. Regarding the presumed hereditary cases, we cannot distinguish with these data between a common recessive trait with about 40% penetrance, a rare dominant trait with about 20% penetrance or genetic heterogeneity.

The frequency of hearing loss of all kinds was significantly greater in white isolated cases than in the white non-malformed group. This was not the case for blacks although the frequency in black isolated cases was twice that found in the black non-malformed group. There was no increased risk of hearing loss in familial cases of either race. The frequency of speech production anomalies (disarticulation) in the absence of hearing loss, mental retardation, and speech mechanism pathology in white isolated cases was significantly greater than that in the white non-malformed group. This was not so for black isolated cases or for familial cases of either race.

References

Aase JM, Tegtmeier RE: Microtia in New Mexico: Evidence for multifactorial causation. In "Numerical Taxonomy of Birth Defects and Polygenic Disorders." BD:OAS XIII(3A):113-116, 1977.*

Adam A: Genetic diseases among Jews. In Ramot B (ed): "Genetic Polymorphisms and Diseases in Man." New York: Academic Press, 1974, pp 257-266.

Altmann F: Malformations of the auricle and the external auditory meatus. A critical review. Arch Otolaryngol 54:115-139, 1951.

Ampola MG: A new familial malformation syndrome. In "Malformation Syndromes." BD:OAS X(7):129-135, 1974.

Anson BJ, Donaldson JA: "Surgical Anatomy of the Temporal Bone and Ear." 2nd Ed. Philadelphia: WB Saunders, 1973.

Armendares S, Antillon F, del Castillo V, Jimenez M: A newly recognized inherited syndrome of dwarfism, craniosynostosis, retinitis pigmentosa and multiple congenital malformations. In "New Chromosomal and Malformation Syndromes." BD:OAS XI(5):49-53, 1975.

Arnold W, Weidauer H, Seelig HP: Experimenteller Beweis einer gemeinsamen Antigenizitat zwischen Innenohr und Niere. Arch Otorhinolaryngol (NY) 212:99-117, 1976.

Aronsohn RS, Batsakis JG, Rice DH, Work WP: Anomalies of the first branchial cleft. Arch Otolaryngol 102:737-740, 1976.

Bailleul JP, Lebersa C, Laude M: Surdité et fistules auriculaires congenitales familiales. Pediatrie 27:739-747, 1972.

Barr M, Burdi AR: Potter syndrome with and without fetal renal abnormality. Teratology 13:16A, 1976.

Beals RK: Auriculo-osteodysplasia. A syndrome of multiple osseous dysplasia, ear anomaly, and short stature. J Bone Joint Surg 49-A:1541-1550, 1967.

Benirschke K: Placental causes of maldevelopment. In Berry CL, Poswillo DE (eds): "Teratology. Trends and Applications." Berlin: Springer-Verlag, 1975, pp 148-164.

Bennett D: The T-locus of the mouse. Cell 6:441-454, 1975.

Bergsma D (ed): "Birth Defects Atlas and Compendium." The National Foundation-March of Dimes. Baltimore: Williams & Wilkins, 1973.

Bhaskar SN, Bernier JL: Histogenesis of branchial cysts: A report of 468 cases. Am J Pathol 35:407-423, 1959.

Bixler D, Christian JC, Gorlin RJ: Hypertelorism, microtia and facial clefting. A newly described inherited syndrome. Am J Dis Child 118:495-500, 1969.

Black FO, Myers EN, Rorke LB: Aplasia of the first and second branchial arches. Arch Otolaryngol 98:124-128, 1973.

Blair, JD: Trisomy C and cystic dysplasia of kidneys, liver and pancreas. In "Cytogenetics, Environment and Malformation." BD:OAS XII(5):139-149, 1976.

Borgaonkar DS, Lacassie YE, Stoll C: Usefulness of chromosome catalog in delineating new syndromes. Ibid pp 87-95.

Bourguet J, Mazeas R, Lettuerou: De l'atteinte de deux premiers arcs branchiaux. Rev Oto-neuro-ophtal 38:161-175, 1966.

*BD:OAS refers to Birth Defects: Original Article Series published by or for The National Foundation—March of Dimes.

Brander T: Zur Kenntnis der Ätiologie der Ohranhänge. Acta Derm Venereol (Stockh) 20:211-222, 1939.
Broman SH, Nichols PL, Kennedy WA: "Preschool IQ. Prenatal and Early Developmental Correlates." Hillsdale, NJ: Lawrence Erlbaum Associates, 1975.
Broome DL, Ebbin AJ, Jung AL, Feinauer LR, Madsen M: Aberrant tissue bands and craniofacial defects. In "Cytogenetics Environment and Malformation Syndromes." BD:OAS XII(5): 65-79, 1976.
Buchta R, Viseskul C, Gilbert EF, Santo GE, Opitz JM: Familial bilateral renal agenesis and hereditary renal adysplasia. Z Kinderheilkd 115:111-129, 1973.
Carson M, Reid M: Warfarin and fetal abnormality. Lancet 1: 1356, 1976.
Cavalli-Sforza LL, Bodmer WF: "The Genetics of Human Populations." San Francisco: WH Freeman and Company, 1971, pp 513-565.
Center for Disease Control: Congenital Malformations Surveillance Report April 1974-March 1975, Issued September 1975.
Chung CS, Brown KS: Family studies of early childhood deafness ascertained through the Clark School for the deaf. Am J Hum Genet 22:630-644, 1970.
Cohen MM: On the nature of syndrome delineation. Acta Genet Med Gemellol (Roma) 26:103-119, 1977.
Congdon ED, Rowhanavongse S, Varamisara P: Human congenital auricular and juxta-auricular fossae, sinuses and scars (including the so-called aural and auricular fistulae) and the bearing of their anatomy upon the theories of their genesis. Am J Anat 51:439-459, 1932.
Connon FE: The inheritance of ear pits in six generations of a family. J Hered 32:413-414, 1941.
Conway H, Wagner KJ: Congenital anomalies of the head and neck as reported on birth certificates in New York City, 1952 to 1962 (inclusive). Plast Reconstr Surg 36:71-79, 1965.
Corliss CE: "Patten's Human Embryology. Elements of Clinical Development." New York: McGraw-Hill, 1976.
Crow JF: Problems in ascertainment in the analysis of family data. In Neel JV, Shaw MW, Schull WJ (eds): "Epidemiology and Genetics of Chronic Diseases." Washington, DC: US Dept of Health, Education and Welfare, 1965, pp 23-41.
Czeizel A, Tusnady G: A family study on cleft lip with or without cleft palate and posterior cleft palate in Hungary. Hum Hered 22:405-416, 1972.
DiSaia PJ: Pregnancy and delivery of a patient with a Starr-Edwards mitral valve prosthesis. Obstet Gynecol 28:469-472, 1966.
Deol MS: Inherited diseases of the inner ear in man in the light of studies on the mouse. J Med Genet 5:137-158, 1968.
Dunn PM: Congenital postural deformities. Br Med Bull 32:71-76, 1976.
Edelman GM: Surface modulation in cell recognition and cell growth. Science 192:218-226, 1976.
Edmonds HW, Keeler CE: Natural "ear-ring" holes. Inherited sinuses of the ear lobe. J Hered 31:507-510, 1940.
Elandt-Johnson RC: "Probability Models and Statistical Methods in Genetics." New York: John Wiley & Sons, 1971, pp 474-479.
Elejalde BR, Giraldo C, Jimenez R, Gilbert EF: Acrocephalopolydactylous dysplasia. In "New Syndromes." BD:OAS XIII(3B):53-67, 1977.
Ellwood LC, Winter ST, Dar H: Familial microtia with meatal atresia in two sibships. J Med Genet 5:289-291, 1968.
Emerson DJ: Congenital malformation due to attempted abortion with aminopterin. Am J Obstet Gynecol 84:356-357, 1962.
Emery AEH: "Methodology in Medical Genetics." Edinburgh: Churchill Livingstone, 1976, pp 35-62.

Escher F, Hirt H: Dominant hereditary conductive deafness through lack of incus-stapes junction. Acta Otolaryngol (Stockh) 65:25-32, 1968.
Ewing MR: Congenital sinuses of the external ear. J Laryng 61:18-23, 1946.
Fara M, Chlupackova V, Hrivrakova J: Dismorphia oto-facio-cervicalis familiaris. Acta Chir Plast (Praha) 9:255-268, 1967.
Fedrick J: Epilepsy and pregnancy: A report from the Oxford record linkage study. Br Med J 2:442-448, 1973.
Fitch N, Srolovitz H: Severe renal dysgenesis produced by a dominant gene. Am J Dis Child 130:1356-1357, 1976.
Fourman F, Fourman J: Hereditary deafness in family with ear pits (fistula auris congenita). Br Med J 2:1354-1356, 1955.
Fraser FC: The multifactorial/threshold concept — uses and misuses. Teratology 14:267-280, 1976.
Fraser FC, Ling D, Clogg D: Deafness, ear pits, branchial fistulae and renal anomalies (Abstract). Am J Hum Genet 29:43A, 1977.
German J, Lowal A, Ehlers KH: Trimethadione and human teratogenesis. Teratology 349-362, 1970.
Gluecksohn-Waelsch S: Genetic control of mammalian differentiation. "Genetics Today," Vol. 2, Proceedings of the XI International Congress of Genetics. The Hague, Netherlands, 1963.
Goldberg MJ, Pashayan HM: Hallux syndactyly-ulnar polydactyly-abnormal ear lobes: A new syndrome. In "Cytogenetics, Environment and Malformation Syndromes." BD:OAS XII(5):255-266, 1976.
Gorlin RJ, Pindborg JJ, Cohen MM: "Syndromes of the Head and Neck." New York: McGraw-Hill, 1976.
Grabb, WC: The first and second branchial arch syndrome. Plast Reconstr Surg 36:485-508, 1965.
Gualandri V: Ricerche genetiche sulla fistula auris congenita. Acta Genet Med Gemellol (Roma) 18:51-68, 1969.
Guenther WC: "Concepts of Probability." New York: McGraw-Hill, 1968, pp 355-360.
Haldane JBS: The estimation and significance of the logarithm of a ratio of frequencies. Ann Hum Genet 20:309-311, 1956.
Hall JG: Embryopathy associated with oral anticoagulant therapy. In "Cytogenetics, Environment and Malformation Syndromes." BD:OAS XII(5):33-37, 1976.
Hanson JW, Freeman MG: Aberrant tissue bands and multiple congenital defects: An epidemiologic assessment. In "New Chromosomal and Malformation Syndromes." (Abstract) BD:OAS XI(5):329, 1975.
Hanson JW, Smith DW: The fetal hydantoin syndrome. J Pediatr 87:285-291, 1975.
Hanson JW, Myrianthopoulos NC, Harvey MAS, Smith DW: Risks to the offspring of women treated with hydantoin anticonvulsant, with emphasis on the fetal hydantoin syndrome. J Pediatr 89:662-668, 1976.
Harada O, Ishii H: The condition of the auditory ossicles in microtia. Plast Reconstr Surg 50:48-53, 1972.
Harrod MJ, Keele DK, Howard J: A syndrome of craniofacial, digital, and genital anomalies. In "New Syndromes." BD:OAS XIII(3B):111-115, 1977.
Herrmann J, Pallister PD, Tiddy W, Opitz JM: The KBG syndrome — a syndrome of short stature, characteristic facies, mental retardation, macrodontia and skeletal anomalies. In "New Chromosomal and Malformation Syndromes." BD:OAS XI(5):7-18, 1975.
Hilson D: Malformation of ears as a sign of malformation of the genito-urinary tract. Br Med J 2:785-789, 1957.
Hollister DW, Klein SH, DeJager HJ, Lachman RS, Rimoin DL: The lacrimo-auriculo-dento-digital syndrome. J Pediatr 83:438-444, 1973.

Hook EB, Marden PM, Reiss NP, Smith DW: Some aspects of the epidemiology of human minor birth defects and morphological variants in a completely ascertained newborn population (Madison Study). Teratology 13:47-55, 1976.
Hough JVD: Congenital malformations of the middle ear. Arch Otolaryngol 78:335-343, 1963.
Hunter AGW: Inheritance of branchial sinuses and preauricular fistulae. Teratology 9:225-228, 1974.
Jaffe BF: The incidence of ear diseases in the Navajo Indians. Laryngoscope 79:2126-2134, 1969.
Jaffe BF: Pinna anomalies associated with congenital conductive hearing loss. Pediatrics 57:332-341, 1976.
Jenkins R: The occurrence of a skin papillus through four human generations. J Hered 19:174, 1928.
Johnson C: "Introduction to Natural Selection." Baltimore: University Park Press, 1976, pp 11-17.
Johnston MC: The neural crest in abnormalities of the face and brain. In "Morphogenesis and Malformation of Face and Brain." BD:OAS XI(7):1-17, 1975.
Johnston MC, Pratt RM: A developmental approach to teratology. In Berry CL, Poswillo DE (eds): "Teratology. Trends and Applications." Berlin: Springer-Verlag, 1975, pp 2-16.
Johnston MC, Bhakdinaronk A, Reid YC: An expanded role of the neural crest in oral and pharyngeal development. In Bosma J (ed): "Fourth Symposium on Oral Sensation and Perception: Development in the Fetus and Infant." Washington, DC: US Gov Printing Office, 1975, pp 37-52.
Jones KL: Aberrant tissue bands in face and brain defects. In "Morphogenesis and Malformation of Face and Brain." BD:OAS XI(7):205-206, 1975.
Jones KL, Smith DW, Streissguth AP, Myrianthopoulos NC: Outcome in offspring of chronic alcoholic women. Lancet 1: 1076-1078, 1974.
Karmody CS, Feingold M: Autosomal dominant first and second branchial arch syndrome. A new inherited syndrome? In "Malformation Syndromes." BD:OAS X(7):31-40, 1974.
Kidd KK, Spence MA: Genetic analyses of pyloric stenosis suggesting a specific maternal effect. J Med Genet 13:290-294, 1976.
Kindred JE: Inheritance of a pit in the skin of the left ear. J Hered 12:366-367, 1921.
Konigsmark BW, Gorlin RJ: "Genetic and Metabolic Deafness." Philadelphia: WB Saunders, 1976.
LeDouarin NM: The neural crest in the neck and other parts of the body. In "Morphogenesis and Malformation of Face and Brain." BD:OAS XI(7):19-50, 1975.
Lilienfeld AM: "Foundations of Epidemiology." New York: Oxford University Press, 1976.
Livingstone G: Congenital ear abnormalities due to thalidomide. Proc R Soc Med 58:493-497, 1965.
Marden PM, Smith DW, McDonald MJ: Congenital anomalies in the newborn infant, including minor variations. J Pediatr 64:357-371, 1964.
Martins, AG: Lateral cervical and preauricular sinuses: Their transmission as dominant characters. Br Med J 2:255-256, 1961.
Mayer RJ, Smith RG, Gallo RC: Reverse transcriptase in normal Rhesus monkey placenta. Science 185:864-866, 1974.
McDonough ES: On the inheritance of ear pit (fistula auris congenita) with special reference to twins. J Hered 32:169-170, 1941.
McIntosh R, Merritt KK, Richards MR, Samuels MH, Bellows MT: The incidence of congenital malformations: A study of 5,964 pregnancies. Pediatrics 14:505-522, 1954.
McKusick VA: "Mendelian Inheritance In Man." 5th Ed. Baltimore: The Johns Hopkins University Press, 1978.
McKusick VA: Ethnic distribution of disease in non-Jews. In Ramot B (ed): "Genetic Polymorphisms and Diseases in Man." New York: Academic Press, 1974, pp 249-256.
McLaurin JW, Kloepfer HW, Laguarte JK: Hereditary branchial anomalies and associated hearing impairment. Laryngoscope 76:1277-1288, 1966.

Melnick M, Bixler D, Silk K, Yune H, Nance WE: Autosomal dominant branchiootorenal dysplasia. In "New Chromosomal and Malformation Syndromes." BD:OAS XI(5):121-128, 1975.
Melnick M, Bixler D, Nance WE, Silk K, Yune H: Familial branchio-oto-renal dysplasia: A new addition to the branchial arch syndromes. Clin Genet 9:25-34, 1976.
Melnick M, Shields ED: Allelic restriction: A biologic alternative to multifactorial threshold inheritance. Lancet 1:176-179, 1976.
Melnick M, Shields ED, Bixler D, Conneally PM: Facial clefting: An alternative biologic explanation for its complex etiology. In "Numerical Taxonomy of Birth Defects and Polygenic Disorders." BD:OAS XIII(3A):93-112, 1977.
Melnick M, Eastman JR: Autosomal dominant maxillofacial dysostosis. In "New Syndromes." BD:OAS XIII(3B):39-44, 1977.
Melnick M, Hodes ME, Nance WE, Yune H, Sweeney A: Branchio-oto-renal dysplasia and branchio-oto-dysplasia: Two distinct autosomal dominant disorders. Clin Genet 13:425-442, 1978.
Meltzer HJ: Congenital anomalies due to attempted abortion with 4-aminopteroglutamic acid. JAMA 161:1253, 1956.
Mengel MC, Konigsmark BW, Berlin CI, McKusick VA: Conductive hearing loss and malformed low-set ears, as a possible recessive syndrome. J Med Genet 6:14-21, 1969.
Merz T: Radiation-induced malformations in man. In "Cytogenetics, Environment and Malformation Syndromes." BD:OAS XII(5):19-22, 1976.
Milunsky A, Graef JW, Gaynor MF: Methotrexate-induced congenital malformations. J Pediatr 72:790-795, 1968.
Monson RR, Rosenberg L, Hartz SC, Shapiro S, Heinonen OP, Slone D: Diphenylhydantoin and selected congenital malformations. N Engl J Med 289:1049-1052, 1973.
Moore KL: "The Developing Human. Clinically Oriented Embryology." Philadelphia: WB Saunders, 1973.
Morton NE: Genetic tests under incomplete ascertainment. Am J Hum Genet 11:1-16, 1959.
Muckle TJ: Hereditary branchial defects in Hampshire family. Br Med J 1:1297-1299, 1961.
Myrianthopoulos NC: "Congenital Malformations in Twins: Epidemiologic Survey." BD:OAS XI(8), 1975.
Myrianthopoulos NC: Epidemiology of central nervous system malformations. In Vinken PJ, Bruyn GW (eds): "Handbook of Clinical Neurology" Vol 30. Amsterdam: North-Holland Publishing Co, 1977.
Myrianthopoulos NC, Chung CS: "Congenital Malformations in Singletons: Epidemiologic Survey." BD:OAS X(11), 1974.
Myrianthopoulos NC, French KS: An application of the U.S. Bureau of the Census socioeconomic index to a large, diversified patient population. Soc Sci Med 2:283-299, 1968.
Naunton RF, Valvassori GE: Inner ear anomalies: Their association with atresia. Laryngoscope 78: 1041-1049, 1968.
Nelson MM, Forfar JO: Congenital abnormalities at birth: Their association in the same patient. Dev Med Child Neurol 11:3-16, 1969.
Newby HA: "Audiology." 2nd Ed. New York: Appleton-Century-Crofts, 1964, pp 95-99.
Nichols MM: Fetal anomalies following maternal trimethadione ingestion. J Pediatr 82:885-886, 1973.
Nishimura H, Okamoto N: "Sequential Atlas of Human Congenital Malformations." Baltimore: University Park Press, 1976.
Nishimura H, Tanimura T: "Clinical Aspects of the Teratogenicity of Drugs." Amsterdam: Excerpta Medica, 1976.
Niswander KR, Gordon M: "The Women and Their Pregnancies." Bethesda: National Institutes of Health, 1972.
Noden DM: The migratory behavior of neural crest cells. In Bosma J (ed): "Fourth Symposium on Oral Sensation and Perception: Development in the Fetus and Infant." Washington, DC: US Gov Printing Office, 1975, pp 9-36.

Noel B, Quack B, Rethore MO: Partial deletions and trisomies of chromosome 13: Mapping of bands associated with particular malformations. Clin Genet 9:593-602, 1976.

Ostmann P: Die Missbildungen des äusseren Ohres unter den Voksschulkindern des Kreises Marburg. Arch Ohrenheilk 58:168-170, 1903.

"Paris Conference. Standardization in human cytogenetics." The National Foundation-March of Dimes. BD:OAS VIII(7), 1972.

Pena SDJ, Shokeir MHK: Syndrome of camptodactyly, multiple ankyloses, facial anomalies and pulmonary hypoplasia – further delineation and evidence for autosomal recessive inheritance. In "Cytogenetics, Environment and Malformation Syndromes." BD:OAS XII(5):201-208, 1976.

Penrose LS: The genetical background of common diseases. Acta Genet 4:257-265, 1953.

Penrose LS: Parental age and mutation. Lancet 2:312-313, 1955.

Peterson DM, Schimke RN: Hereditary cup-shaped ears and the Pierre Robin syndrome. J Med Genet 5:52-55, 1968.

Poswillo D: Observations of fetal posture and causal mechanisms of deformity of palate, mandible and limbs. J Dent Res 45:584-596, 1966.

Poswillo D: The pathogenesis of the first and second branchial arch syndrome. Oral Surg 35:302-328, 1973.

Poswillo D: Otomandibular deformity: Pathogenesis as a guide to reconstruction. J Maxillofac Surg 2:64-72, 1974.

Poswillo D: Hemorrhage in development of the face. In "Morphogenesis and Malformation of Face and Brain." BD:OAS XI(7):61-81, 1975.

Poswillo D: Mechanisms and pathogenesis of malformations. Br Med Bull 32:59-64, 1976.

Poswillo D, Nunnerly H, Sopher D, Keith J: Hyperthermia as a teratogenic agent. Ann R Coll Surg Engl 55:171-174, 1974.

Potter EL: A hereditary ear malformation transmitted through five generations. J Hered 28:255-258, 1937.

Powell HR, Ekert H: Methotrexate-induced congenital malformations. Med J Aust 2:1076-1077, 1971.

Proctor B, Proctor C: Congenital lesions of the head and neck. Otolaryngol Clin North Am 3:221-248, 1970.

Qazi QH, Masakawa A: Altered sex ratio in fetal alcohol syndrome. Lancet 2:42, 1976.

Quelprud T: Ear pit and its inheritance. Fistula auris congenita, described in 1864, still a genetical and embryological puzzle. J Hered 31:379-384, 1940.

Quick CA, Fish A, Brown C: The relationship between cochlea and kidney. Laryngoscope 83:1469-1482, 1973.

Rao CR: "Advanced Statistical Methods in Biometric Research." New York: John Wiley & Sons, 1952, pp 210-214.

Ride L: cited in Altmann (1951).

Rogers BO: Microtic, lop, cup and protruding ears: Four directly inheritable deformities? Plast Reconstr Surg 41:208-231, 1968.

Rohlf FJ, Sokal RR: "Statistical Tables." San Francisco: WH Freeman and Company, 1969, pp 152-156.

Ross RB: Discussion. In "Morphogenesis and Malformation of Face and Brain." BD:OAS XI(7):81, 1975.

Rowley PT: Familial hearing loss associated with branchial fistulas. Pediatrics 44:978-985, 1969.

Ruttin E: Zur Frage der Fistula auris congenita und der Aurikularanhänge. Wien med Wschr 77:1019-1020, 1927.

Selkirk TE: Fistula auris congenita. Am J Dis Child 49:431-447, 1935.

Shapiro LR, Duncan PA, Farnsworth PB, Lefkowitz M: Congenital microcephaly, hiatus hernia and nephrotic syndrome: An autosomal recessive syndrome. In "Cytogenetics, Environment and Malformation Syndromes." BD:OAS XII(5):275-278, 1976.

Shaw EB, Steinbach HL: Aminopterin-induced fetal malformation. Survival of infant after attempted abortion. Am J Dis Child 115:477-482, 1968.

Shenoi PM: Wildervanck's syndrome. J Laryngol Otol 86:1121-1135, 1972.

Shepard TH: "Catalog of Teratogenic Agents." Baltimore: The John Hopkins University Press, 1973.

Sherman S, Hall BD: Warfarin and fetal abnormality. Lancet 1: 692, 1976.

Siemens HW: Zur Kenntnis der sogenannten Ohr-und Halsanhänge (branchiogene Knorpelmaeir). Arch Derm Syph (Berl) 132:186-205, 1921.

Simpkiss M, Lowe A: Congenital abnormalities in the African newborn. Arch Dis Child 36:404-406, 1961.

Smith DW: "Recognizable Patterns of Human Malformation." 2nd Ed. Philadelphia: WB Saunders, 1976.

Smithells RW: Environmental teratogens of man. Br Med Bull 32:27-33, 1976.

Sokal RR, Rohlf FJ: "Biometry." San Francisco: WH Freeman and Company, 1969.

Speidel BD, Meadow SR: Maternal epilepsy and abnormalities of the fetus and newborn. Lancet 2: 839-843, 1972.

Stannus HS: Congenital anomalies in a native African race. Biometrika 10:1-24, 1914.

Stark RB: Development of the face. Gynecol Obstet 92:891–900, 1973.

Stevenson AC, Johnston HA, Stewart MIP, Golding DR: Congenital malformations. A report of a study of series of consecutive births in 24 centers. Bull WHO 34(Suppl):1-127, 1966a.

Stevenson AC, Johnston HA, Golding DR, Stewart MIP: "Comparative Study of Congenital Malformations. Basic Tabulations in Respect of Consecutive Post 28-week Births Recorded in the Cooperative Centers." Oxford: Medical Research Council, Population Genetic Research Unit, 1966b.

Stevenson SS, Worcester J, Rice RG: 667 congenitally malformed infants and associated gestational characteristics. Pediatrics 6:37-50, 1950.

Stiles KA: The inheritance of pitted ear. J Hered 36:53-61, 1945.

Streeter GL: Focal deficiencies in fetal tissues and their relations to intrauterine amputations. Contr Embryol Carneg Instn 22:1-44, 1930.

Thiersch JB: Therapeutic abortions with a folic acid antagonist, 4-aminopterylglutamic acid (4-amino PGA) administered by the oral route. Am J Obstet Gynecol 63:1298-1304, 1952.

Torpin RC: "Malformations Caused by Amnion Rupture During Gestation." Springfield: Charles C Thomas, 1968, p 180.

Townes PL, Brocks ER: Hereditary syndrome of imperforate anus with hand, foot, and ear anomalies. J Pediatr 81:321-326, 1972.

Tuchmann-Duplessis H, David G, Haegel P: "Illustrated Human Embryology." Vol 1, "Embryogenesis." New York: Springer-Verlag, 1972.

Tuchmann-Duplessis H, Haegel P: "Illustrated Human Embryology." Vol 2, "Organogenesis." New York: Springer-Verlag, 1974.

Tuchmann-Duplessis H, Auroux M, Haegel P: "Illustrated Human Embryology." Vol 3, "Nervous System and Endocrine Glands." New York: Springer-Verlag, 1974.

Villumsen AL: "Environmental Factors In Congenital Malformations: A prospective study of 9006 human pregnancies." Copenhagen: FADLs Forlag, 1970.

Warkany J: "Congenital Malformations." Chicago: Year Book Medical Publishers, 1971.

Warkany J, Beaudry PH, Hornstein S: Attempted abortion with aminopterin (4-aminopteroylglutamic acid). Am J Dis Child 97:274-281, 1959.
Wheeler CE, Shaw RF, Cawley EP: Branchial anomalies in three generations of one family. Arch Dermatol 77:715-719, 1958.
Whitney DD: Three generations of ear pits. J Hered 30:323-324, 1939.
Whitson TC: Anomaly of the first branchial cleft. Plast Reconstr Surg 42:595-597, 1968.
Wildervanck LS: Hereditary malformations of the ear in three generations. Acta Otolaryngol 54:533-560, 1962.
Winter JSD, Kohn G, Mellman WJ, Wagner S: A familial syndrome of renal, genital and middle ear anomalies. J Pediatr 72:88-93, 1968.
Zackai EH, Mellman WJ, Neiderer B, Hanson JW: The fetal trimethadione syndrome. J Pediatr 87:280-284, 1975.

Index

Alcohol, 48
Aminopterin, 49–50
Aminopterin syndrome, 50
Amniotic fluid, 18–19, 47
Anotia, 12, 22
Anticonvulsants, 49
Appendages, auricular, 15
Auricular deformations. *See* Deformations, ear
Auriculo-osteodysplasia, 28, 122

Birth order, 99
Birthweight, low, 107
Bixler syndrome, 28, 122
Branchial region
  normal morphogenesis of, 1–7
  See also First and second branchial arch syndrome
Branchio-oto dysplasia, 27, 122
Branchio-oto-renal dysplasia, 23–27, 122

Chromosomal aberrations, 44–45
Collaborative Perinatal Project (NCPP) study, 55–128
Congenital malformations. *See* Malformations, congenital
Cryptotia, 14, 22
Cup ears, 13, 122
Cysts, lateral cervical, 17–18

Deformations, ear, 18–19, 121, 122
Diseases during pregnancy, 101
Drugs, maternal use of, 103–4
Dysmorphogenesis, ear, 11; *See also* Deformations, ear; Malformations, congenital ear; Morphogenesis

Environmental agents, 45–51, 95–105, 120
Environment-gene interaction, 51, 104–5
Epidemiology, ear malformation, 31–40, 61–63
Escher-Hirt syndrome, 28, 122
Etiology, ear malformation, 41–51, 72–74
Eustachian tube malformation, 17

Fetal membranes, 46–47
Fetus deformation, 18–19
First and second branchial arch syndrome, 19–21, 40, 96–99, 124
Fistulas
  anomalies of communicating branchial, 17
  auricular, 14–15

Gene-environment interaction, 51, 104–5
Genetic counseling, 119
Genetics and ear malformations, 41–51, 63–65, 83–93, 118–19

Hearing loss, 110–13, 127–28
Hemorrhage hypothesis, 96–99

Incus malformations, 17
Infectious agents, 47, 101
Intelligence, 108–9

LADD syndrome, 28, 122
Laterality, 39, 75, 117
Lobule anomalies, 14
Lop ears, 13, 122

Macrotia, 15–16
Malformations, congenital ear,
    11–29
    associated with other malformations,
        39–40, 121, 123
    branchial cleft, 17–18, 31–51, 117,
        122–24
    and environmental agents, 95–105,
        120
    epidemiology, 31–40, 61–63
    etiology, 41–51, 72–74
    external ear, 12–16, 31–51, 107,
        117, 122–24
    familial vs isolated, 74–75, 78–79
    and genetics, 41–51, 63–65, 83–93,
        118–19
    institutional variations in, 78–82
    isolated, 74–75, 78–79, 107
    laterality of, 39, 75, 117
    middle ear, 16–17
    nonsyndromic cases, 75–77
    pouch anomalies, 17–18
    and racial distribution, 78–82,
        117–18, 127–28
    sex distribution, 37–39, 77–78, 127
    syndromes, 19–29, 120–21
    See also Deformation, ear
Malleus malformation, 17
Mandibulofacial dysostosis, 21–22, 122
Meatus, atresia of external auditory, 14
Mengel syndrome, 28, 122
Methotrexate, 49–50
Methotrexate syndrome, 50
Micro-ear, 16
Microtia, 12, 122
Microtia-meatal atresia-conductive
    hearing loss syndrome, 28, 122
Middle ear
    anomalies, 124
    normal morphogenesis of, 8–10

Morphogenesis
    of branchial region, 1–7
    of external ear, 8
    of middle ear, 8–10
    See also Dysmorphogenesis

Oligohydramnios, 19, 122
Otocephaly anomaly, 28
Oto-facio-cervical syndrome, 28, 122
Otomandibular dysostosis, 22–23, 122

Placenta, 46–47
Potter syndrome, 19, 123–24
Pregnancy
    complications in, 103
    disease during, 101
Protruding ears, 13–14, 122

Racial distribution of ear malformations,
    36–37, 40, 78–82, 117–18, 127–28
Radiation, ionizing, 47–48

Sex distribution of ear malformations,
    37–40, 77–78, 127
Sinuses
    anomalies of, 17–18
    auricular, 14–15
Socioeconomic status, 100
Speech production, 114
Stapedial artery, persistent, 17
Stapes, congenital fixation of, 17
Synotia anomaly, 40

Teratogens, 45–51, 107
Thalidomide, 50, 123
Townes-Brock syndrome, 28,
    40, 122
Tympanic cavity anomalies, 16–17

Vaccination, maternal, 102
Warfarin, 50–51

BOOKS PUBLISHED BY ALAN R. LISS, INC.
FOR THE NATIONAL FOUNDATION

BIRTH DEFECTS: ORIGINAL ARTICLE SERIES

1975 — Volume XI

No. 7 **Morphogenesis and Malformation of Face and Brain,** Daniel Bergsma and Jan Langman, *Editors*

1976 — Volume XII

No. 1 **Cancer and Genetics,** Daniel Bergsma, R. Neil Schimke, Robert L. Summitt, and David J. Harris, *Editors*

No. 3 **The Eye and Inborn Errors of Metabolism,** Daniel Bergsma, Anthony J. Bron and Edward Cotlier, *Editors*

No. 4 **Developmental Disabilities: Psychologic and Social Implications,** Daniel Bergsma and Ann E. Pulver, *Editors*

No. 5 **Cytogenetics, Environment and Malformation Syndromes,** Daniel Bergsma and R. Neil Schimke, *Editors*

No. 6 **Growth Problems and Clinical Advances,** Daniel Bergsma and R. Neil Schimke, *Editors*

No. 8 **Iron Metabolism and Thalassemia,** Daniel Bergsma, Anthony Cerami, Charles M. Peterson, and Joseph H. Graziano, *Editors*

1977 — Volume XIII

No. 1 **Morphogenesis and Malformation of the Limb,** Daniel Bergsma and Widukind Lenz, *Editors*

No. 2 **Morphogenesis and Malformation of the Genital System,** Richard J. Blandau and Daniel Bergsma, *Editors*

No. 3 **Annual Review of Birth Defects, 1976,** Daniel Bergsma and R. Brian Lowry, *Editors*
Proceedings of the 1976 Vancouver Birth Defects Conference.
Published in 4 volumes:
- 3A **Numerical Taxonomy of Birth Defects** *and* **Polygenic Disorders**
- 3B **New Syndromes**
- 3C **Natural History of Specific Birth Defects**
- 3D **Embryology and Pathogenesis** *and* **Prenatal Diagnosis**

No. 5 **Urinary System Malformations in Children,** Daniel Bergsma and John W. Duckett, *Editors*

No. 6 **Trends and Teaching in Clinical Genetics,** Daniel Bergsma, Frederick Hecht, Gerald H. Prescott, and Joan H. Marks, *Editors*

1978 — Volume XIV

No. 1 **Genetic Effects on Aging,** Daniel Bergsma and David E. Harrison, *Editors*

No. 2 **The Molecular Basis of Cell-Cell Interaction,** Richard A. Lerner and Daniel Bergsma, *Editors*

No. 3 **The Genetics of Hand Malformations,** *by* Samia A. Temtamy and Victor A. McKusick

No. 5   **Neurochemical and Immunologic Components in Schizophrenia,** Daniel Bergsma and Allan L. Goldstein, *Editors*

No. 6   **Annual Review of Birth Defects, 1977,** Robert L. Summitt and Daniel Bergsma, *Editors*
Proceedings of the 1977 Memphis Birth Defects Conference. Published in 3 volumes:
- 6A   **Cell Surface Factors, Immune Deficiencies, Twin Studies**
- 6B   **Recent Advances** *and* **New Syndromes**
- 6C   **Sex Differentiation** *and* **Chromosomal Abnormalities**

No. 7   **Morphogenesis and Malformation of the Cardiovascular System,** Glenn C. Rosenquist and Daniel Bergsma, *Editors*